Numeracy in Nursing and Healthcare

Calculations and Practice

Pearl Shihab BSc, MSc, RN, RM, RNT

Former Senior Tutor in Nursing Studies,
European Institute of Health and Medical Sciences,
University of Surrey

PEARSON
Education

Harlow, England • London • New York • Boston • San Francisco • Toronto
Sydney • Tokyo • Singapore • Hong Kong • Seoul • Taipei • New Delhi
Cape Town • Madrid • Mexico City • Amsterdam • Munich • Paris • Milan

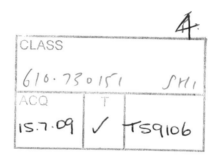

Pearson Education Limited
Edinburgh Gate
Harlow
Essex CM20 2JE
England

and Associated Companies throughout the world

Visit us on the World Wide Web at:
www.pearsoned.co.uk

First published 2009

ISBN: 978-0-273-72074-4

British Library Cataloguing-in-Publication Data
A catalogue record for this book is available from the British Library.

Library of Congress Cataloging-in-Publication Data
Shihab, Pearl.
  Numeracy in nursing and healthcare : calculations and practice /
  Pearl Shihab.
    p. ; cm.
  Includes bibliographical references and index.
  ISBN 978-0-273-72074-4 (pbk.)
 1. Nursing—Mathematics. 2. Pharmaceutical arithmetic. I. Title.
  [DNLM: 1. Mathematics—Nurses' Instruction. 2. Drug Dosage
Calculations—Nurses' Instruction. QT 35 S555n 2009]
  RT68.S55 2009
  610.73—dc22

                                         2009000269

10 9 8 7 6 5 4 3 2 1
13 12 11 10 09

Typeset in 9.5/13 Din Regular by 73.
Printed in Great Britain by Henry Ling Limited at the Dorset Press, Dorchester.

The publisher's policy is to use paper manufactured from sustainable forests.

Contents

8 Common clinical measurements 145

Charting, charting and more charting

9 Physiological measurements 171

Blood, but no sweat and tears

10 Statistics and reading research articles 185

No ostriches here, please

Appendices

Introduction

The purpose of this book is first to develop your basic arithmetic skills and then apply that knowledge to areas of your programme where you will meet numbers. Emphasis is on safety in calculating drug doses but the range is widened to cover clinical and physiological measurements.

Arithmetic is a language using symbols and numbers instead of letters. Fortunately, it is not totally foreign, although you may think differently! We use numbers every day, whether to see the number of the bus we need to take us to the shops or the number of pounds and pence we have to pay for our purchases when we get there.

If you looked at the price tag on an MP3 player and found that it said twenty-seven pounds and ninety-nine pence rather than £27.99 you would be very surprised. Numbers make this type of information much quicker to understand.

However, some people panic if they are asked to use these same numbers in a different way. I hope by using this book in a way that suits you that you will be as confident in using the language of arithmetic as you are in using letters to make words and sentences.

When a child learns to speak or you learn a foreign language, there are certain rules that must be learned, but sometimes (or often) the rule doesn't apply and we make mistakes. Listen to small children: they learn to speak by listening and picking up the rules. For example, the use of the ending –ed on a verb usually means that it happened in the past, such as when we say, 'I walked up the hill'. It is a very common way of indicating past tense. Children hear this form so often they start to form their own versions of verbs, applying what they have learned. They will say such things as 'I goed to playschool' – logical, but the rule does not apply. How confusing is that?

In arithmetic, the rules are much tighter and do not change, so if you follow the rules, then you'll be fine.

Making the book work for you

There are a number of check points in the chapters so that you can make sure that you have really got to grips with the material. If you know it all already, just double check by doing the starting point questions at the beginning of each section.

You are encouraged to do the examples in the first chapter without a calculator. It is all too easy to input the wrong information and not realise. It is better that you know the approximate answer so that you can spot errors. In any case, mental arithmetic is gym for the brain, keeping it in good working order. Just look at the number of games there are for consoles and hand-held computers. It just proves that maths can be fun.

Writing down a sum is fine if it helps you, but use your head to do the calculation.

Most of the chapters are divided into sections that start with a self-assessment. If you do not have all the questions right, you will have to decide whether you need to work through the whole section or the parts that you feel you need to revise. Immediately after each topic, there are some examples for you to try to give you confidence that you have thoroughly understood the material. If you feel in need of more practice, there are more examples at the end of the chapter.

The most important thing is that you use the book in the best way for you. Use a notebook to keep track of your progress by writing down your answers and any points you don't understand.

Don't think that you are on your own. Form study groups and help each other, look at websites and talk to your lecturers and mentors.

A few key books are suggested so that you can look at topics in more detail. Books are a very individual choice, so look at different books of the same level.

Throughout the book there are a number of symbols which help to guide you through each chapter.

YOUR STARTING POINT

Not everyone using this book will be starting off at the same point. The early chapters start off gently so that you can surprise yourself with how much you really know and gain confidence.

If you are generally confident with your ability, you can identify any weak areas and then go to the appropriate part of the chapter to brush up on them.

You do not need to work through the whole chapter – just follow the directions at the end of the test.

TIME TO TRY

These tests are put in after each new topic so that you can find out how much you have learned (or already knew). There is a further similar test at the end of the chapter if you feel the need for more practice.

APPLYING THE THEORY

These are snippets to help put the content of the chapter into context, either in the clinical setting or in everyday life. It is useful if you can find examples of your own when you are in the clinical areas.

KEY POINTS

A short bullet-point list of the important issues that you need to remember.

LOOK OUT

Potential hazards that you may not be aware of as a student.

This symbol alerts you to how the current topic is related to or supported by material in other parts of the book.

 ## RUNNING WORDS

This is a list of terms that were introduced in the chapter and with which you should be familiar. Write them in a notebook and define them in your own words, then go back through the chapter to check the accuracy.

 ## WHAT DID YOU LEARN?

This is a quiz that covers the content of the chapter. You can then go back to a section of the chapter if you are unsure of your answer.

 ## WEB RESOURCES

Many of these sites have interactive material to give you a different perspective on the material. There are various levels of activity in many of the sites, so you can choose your own starting point. Some sites are just for fun, although they make some serious points.

Acknowledgements

We would like to thank the reviewers for their comments:

Maggie Davidson, University of Hertfordshire
Lynne Henshaw, Middlesex University
James Richardson, Curriculum Support Manager, Directorate of Nursing, The University of Liverpool

We are grateful to the following for permission to reproduce copyright material:

Figures

Figure 3.1a from Ohaus Corporation; Figure 3.3 from *Get ready for A&P*, 1st ed., Pearson Education (Garrett, Lori K. 2007) Figure 2.7b, p. 78; Copyright 2007 by Pearson Education Inc. Reprinted by permission.; Figure 8.8 from www.merck.com/media/mmhe2/figures/MMHE_03_022_03_eps.gif, From The Merck Manual of Medical Information – Second Home Edition, edited by Robert S. Porter. Copyright 2007 by Merck & Co., Inc., Whitehouse Station, NJ. Available at: http://www.merck.com/mmhe. Accessed (date).; Visit all of The Merck Manuals free online at www.MerckManuals.com.; Figure 9.1 from http://greenfield.fortunecity.com/rattler/46/haemopoiesis.htm.

Photographs

(Key: b-bottom; c-centre; l-left; r-right; t-top)
P. 63 Fundamental Photographs/Richard Megna (3.2); p. 85 Alamy Images/Profimedia International s.r.o. (4.9/l), Science Photo Library Ltd/Scott Camazine (4.9/r); p. 89 Wellcome Images (4.13); p. 96 Wellcome Images (5.1/t, 5.1/b); p. 100 Wellcome Images (5.2); p. 120 Casio (6.2); p. 129 Mediscan (7.1), Wellcome Images (7.2); p. 130 Baxter Healthcare Ltd (7.3); p. 131 Wellcome Images (7.5); p. 132 Wellcome Images (7.6); p. 137 Baxter Healthcare Ltd (7.7); p. 139 Smiths Medical International (7.8/t, 7.8/b); p. 151 Alamy Images/Mode Images Limited (8.4), Corbis/Chris Collins/Zefa (8.3); p.153 Mediscan (8.5); Wellcome Images (8.6); p. 154 Science Photo Library Ltd/Geoff Kidd (8.7/l/a), Gustoimages (8.7/r/b); p. 156 Clement Clarke International Ltd (8.9); p. 157 Getty Images/Photographers Choice (8.1); p. 177 Alamy Images/Phototake Inc (9.2); p. 180 Mediscan (9.3); p. 184 Science Photo Library Ltd/CRISTINA PEDRAZZINI; p. 211 Clement Clarke International Ltd; p. 212 'Malnutrition Universal Screening Tool' ('MUST') is reproduced here with the kind permission of BAPEN (British Association for Parenteral and Enteral Nutrition).

In some instances we have been unable to trace the owners of copyright material, and we would appreciate any information that would enable us to do so.

Chapter 1

Basic arithmetic skills

The things you don't want to ask about but need to know

You need to be able to add and subtract to complete patient records accurately.

You must be confident with basic arithmetic skills so that you are able to work out correct drug doses to ensure patient safety.

When you have completed this chapter, you should be able to:

- Understand the different ways in which the four basic operations of arithmetic can be written.

- Add and subtract single and multiple columns of figures without a calculator.

- Multiply and divide simple numbers without a calculator.

- Understand how exponents are used to simplify large whole numbers.

- Use 'BODMAS' to work out calculations that involve different types of operation.

- Use a calculator with care.

The language

Table 1.1 shows the symbols that will be used in this chapter – more later! You are probably familiar with them, which is good, but just refresh your memory of these and the rules that apply to them.

Table 1.1

Symbol	Meaning and uses
+	Plus, the sum, altogether, total or increase all indicate that one number is added to the other, e.g. six plus three: 6 + 3. The numbers can be added in any order, the answer is the same. $^+$ can also be used as shorthand for 'positive'; 've' is sometimes added and is written as $^+$ve with the + sign near the top of the ve.
−	Decrease, difference between, reduce by, minus or 'take away' all indicate that the second number is subtracted from the first, e.g. six minus three: 6 − 3. The numbers must *always* be calculated in the order in which they are written. − can also be used as shorthand for 'negative'; 've' is sometimes added and is written as $^-$ve with the − level with the top of the ve.
×	Groups of, lots of, product, sets of or 'times' all indicate that one number is multiplied by the other, e.g. six multiplied by three: 6 × 3. Like addition, it does not matter which number is used first, the answer is the same.
÷ or /	Divide or 'share' – the first number is divided by the second, e.g. six divided by three, 6 ÷ 3 or 6/3, or it can be written as $\frac{6}{3}$. Like subtraction, the numbers must *always* be calculated in the order in which they are written.
=	Is equal to. This is usually the answer to a calculation, e.g. 6 + 3 = 9. If you have six apples and then are given three more, you will have the same number as if you were given all 9 at once.

APPLYING THE THEORY

You will learn more about $^+$ and $^-$ being used to identify positive or negative charges on particles in physiology.

In the UK, blood is identified as being one of four types: A, B, AB or O. In addition, an individual either has or does not have the rhesus factor. The blood is then described as rhesus positive (if the individual has the factor) or negative (if the individual does not) and is written as Rh $^+$ve or Rh $^-$ve.

> **LOOK OUT**
>
> It is important that the correct blood is given to a patient in need of a blood transfusion, so it is safer to write positive or negative in full so that there is no doubt about the rhesus status of the patient or the blood to be transfused.

1.1 ADDITION

YOUR STARTING POINT FOR ADDITION

Without using a calculator, write down the answers to the following questions.

(a) 4 + 5 = _____   (b) 3 + 7 = _____   (c) 12 + 8 = _____

(d) 33 + 67 = _____   (e) 45 + 55 = _____   (f) 47 + 53 = _____

(g) 137 + 21 + 241 = _____   (h) 613 + 13 + 252 = _____

(i) 573 + 37 + 145 = _____   (j) 388 + 133 + 49 = _____

Answers: (a) 9 (b) 10 (c) 20 (d) 100 (e) 100 (f) 100 (g) 399 (h) 878 (i) 755 (j) 570.

If you had these all correct, skip through to Section 1.2 – Subtraction.

Let's start at the beginning – a very good place to start. When you write you begin with ABC, when you sing you begin with doh–ray–me and in maths you start with 123. Each individual figure is a **numeral** but in everyday speech we call them numbers.

Whole numbers are those without fractions, e.g. 7, 21, 155, 3742. They are sometimes called integers.

One of the most important concepts is that of **number bonds**. This is the technical way of adding the numbers together.

Number bonds 1 to 10

0 1 2 3 4 5 6 7 8 9 10

These are the numbers that can be added together to make a total of 10.

Numbers can be added together in any order:

$$0 + 10 = 10$$
$$1 + 9 = 10$$
$$2 + 8 = 10$$
$$3 + 7 = 10$$
$$4 + 6 = 10$$
$$5 + 5 = 10$$
$$6 + 4 = 10$$
$$7 + 3 = 10$$
$$8 + 2 = 10$$
$$9 + 1 = 10$$
$$10 + 0 = 10$$

Can you see a pattern? The first numbers go *up* by 1. The second numbers go *down* by 1.

What is the answer to the following?

$$8 + 2 =$$

$$2 + 8 =$$

Which sum was easier to work out? Why was it easier?

Counting on

0 1 2 3 4 5 6 7 8 9 10

Numbers can be added in any order but it is easier to start with the bigger number and count on. You can also use the line of numbers to check this method if you are not confident. Consider

$$3 + 7 =$$

This can be done as $7 + 3$, keeping 7 in your head and counting on 3.

Hint: Look for the bigger number, keep it in your head and count on.

(a) $2 + 8 =$ _____   (b) $4 + 6 =$ _____

(c) $1 + 9 =$ _____   (d) $3 + 7 =$ _____

You should have got 10 for all these answers.

Now try these. What do you need to make 10?

(a) $9 +$ ___   (b) $5 +$ ___   (c) $7 +$ ___   (d) $10 +$ ___

(e) $2 +$ ___   (f) $1 +$ ___   (g) $3 +$ ___   (h) $0 +$ ___

(i) $4 +$ ___   (j) $6 +$ ___   (k) $8 +$ ___

Answers: (a) 1 (b) 5 (c) 3 (d) 0 (e) 8 (f) 9 (g) 7 (h) 10 (i) 6 (j) 4 (k) 2.

Have you got the idea? If you are confident that you understand the concept of number bonds 1–10, then move on to place value.

Place value

You are now familiar with numbers up to 10 and how they can be added together to make 10. Each time the answer was 10 but the way in which you reached it may have been so automatic that you didn't think about the rule.

Place value is to do with the 'amount a number is worth', depending on where in a line of numbers it is written. If I wrote a cheque for £1, another for £10 and a final one for £100, I would have written 1 three times but in a different place along a line of numbers. Its value goes from one unit, to one 10, then one 100. What a difference a place makes!

Add these numbers together and think about how you achieved the answer:

(a) 5 + 7 = _____   (b) 9 + 4 = _____   (c) 6 + 8 = _____   (d) 7 + 7 = _____

You should have the following answers: (a) 12 (b) 13 (c) 14 (d) 14.

What answer did you get? You probably used the same method as you did for the bonding of the numbers 1 to 10.

In the examples above you had one 10 and some spare units left over, so you put them in the units column. We use a system of counting called base 10 so that when we write 12, it means that we have one lot of 10 and two units. If you were asked to add 15 and 6 your answer would be 21. This means that you have two lots of 10 and one unit left over.

Number bonds 1-20

0 1 2 3 4 5 6 7 8 9 10 11 12 13 14 15 16 17 18 19 20

0 + 20 = 20	6 + 14 = 20	11 + 9 = 20	16 + 4 = 20
1 + 19 = 20	7 + 13 = 20	12 + 8 = 20	17 + 3 = 20
2 + 18 = 20	8 + 12 = 20	13 + 7 = 20	18 + 2 = 20
3 + 17 = 20	9 + 11 = 20	14 + 6 = 20	19 + 1 = 20
4 + 16 = 20	10 + 10 = 20	15 + 5 = 20	20 + 0 = 20
5 + 15 = 20			

Again the pattern here is that the first number increases by one as the second number decreases. Look back at the number bonds 0–10 and you will see the same pattern.

TIME TO TRY

(a) 4 + 16 = _____   (b) 18 + 2 = _____   (c) 9 + 11 = _____

(d) 12 + 8 = _____   (e) 7 + 13 = _____   (f) 19 + 1 = _____

You can add these by counting on as you did with the 0–10 bonds. The answer to all these is 20.

What do you need to add to these numbers to make 20?

(a) 11 + _____   (b) 17 + _____   (c) 6 + _____

(d) 10 + _____   (e) 4 + _____   (f) 18 + _____

(g) 15 + _____   (h) 2 + _____   (i) 13 + _____

Answers: (a) 9 (b) 3 (c) 14 (d) 10 (e) 16 (f) 2 (g) 5 (h) 18 (i) 7.

More about place value

When you had 10 units you wrote 10. Ten lots of 10 overflows the tens column so you write 100, which means that 10 lots of 10 is 100. When you have 10 lots of 100, you write it as 1000 and so on until you run out of energy or ink.

How would you describe, in terms of '10 lots of', 10000?

This number is 10 lots of 1000, i.e. 'ten thousand'. In this case, saying the number aloud gives you the answer!

Number bonds 1 to 100

Look at **Table 1.2**. The numbers in the rows increase by one each time.

What do you notice about the way the numbers in the columns increase? They are bigger than the number above, by 10.

There are 10 rows of 10, so you can use it to count in tens, e.g. start at a number in the top row, say 6, then go down the column and each one is 10 more than the number above: 6, 26, 36, 46 … .

Use the table to help you test your ability to form number bonds with numbers making 100.

What number needs to be added to 73 to make 100?

There are several ways you could solve this problem. The principles that you used to add together for the numbers 0 to 20 can be used for the numbers 0 to 100.

You can count on 74, 75, 76… until you got to 100, but this takes quite a long time and there are many opportunities to miscount.

You can count to 80, then count in tens up to 100 and add the two numbers together to find your answer: 73 to 80 is 7 and 80 to 100 is 20, so your answer to the question is $7 + 20 = 27$.

You can also count in tens from 73 until you get to 93 and then count to 100 from 93. You will then have $20 + 7 = 27$. Miraculously, the same answer!

Table 1.2 Numbers 1 to 100

1	2	3	4	5	6	7	8	9	10
11	12	13	14	15	16	17	18	19	20
21	22	23	24	25	26	27	28	29	30
31	32	33	34	35	36	37	38	39	40
41	42	43	44	45	46	47	48	49	50
51	52	53	54	55	56	57	58	59	60
61	62	63	64	65	66	67	68	69	70
71	72	73	74	75	76	77	78	79	80
81	82	83	84	85	86	87	88	89	90
91	92	93	94	95	96	97	98	99	100

In arithmetic, it doesn't matter how you get the answer as long as it is the right one and you understand the rules that you use. Practise both methods in your head for the following (counting on is not wrong, it just takes a long time with large numbers and there is room for making a mistake).

TIME TO TRY

(a) 23 + 77 = _____   (b) 50 + 50 = _____   (c) 32 + 68 = _____

(d) 45 + 55 = _____   (e) 72 + 28 = _____   (f) 84 + 16 = _____

(g) 65 + 35 = _____   (h) 59 + 41 = _____   (i) 61 + 39 = _____

The answer to all of these is 100.

What needs to be added to these numbers to make 100?

(a) 90 + _____ = 100   (b) 35 + _____ = 100   (c) 64 + _____ = 100

(d) 78 + _____ = 100   (e) 23 + _____ = 100   (f) 85 + _____ = 100

(g) 17 + _____ = 100   (h) 72 + _____ = 100   (i) 56 + _____ = 100

Answers: (a) 10 (b) 65 (c) 36 (d) 22 (e) 77 (f) 15 (g) 83 (h) 28 (i) 44.

Mastered these? Then move on to the next part. If you want more practice, there are further examples at the end of the chapter.

> **KEY POINT**
>
> ● The position of an individual numeral in a number determines its value.

So far, you have added two numbers together. Often, several numbers need to be added to get a total, for instance when you have several items of shopping and need to know whether you have enough money.

Place value is even more important when larger numbers are added together. It is vital that the hundreds, tens and units are placed under each other in the sum. Add 121 + 322 + 55.

```
        H  T  U
        1  2  1
add  +  3  2  2
           5  5
       ─────────
        4  9  8
```

The columns must *always* be added starting from the units column on the right.

First the numbers in the units column are added together: $1 + 2 + 5 = 8$
Next the numbers in the tens column are added together: $2 + 2 + 5 = 9$
Then the numbers in the hundreds column: $3 + 1 = 4$

Look at the difference in the answers below if care is not taken to align the numbers correctly.

```
            H  T  U
            1  2  1
    add  +  3  2  2
            5  5
            ─────────
            9  9  3
```

TIME TO TRY

Use a page in your notebook to set out the sums as in the above examples.

(a) 52 + 230 + 17 = _____   (b) 324 + 241 + 123 = _____

(c) 144 + 211 + 43 = _____   (d) 73 + 410 + 16 = _____

(e) 114 + 612 + 53 = _____   (f) 725 + 142 + 132 = _____

(g) 450 + 114 + 131 = _____   (h) 212 + 412 + 322 = _____

(i) 186 + 12 + 501 = _____   (j) 127 + 21 + 311 = _____

(k) 538 + 20 + 121 = _____   (l) 523 + 51 + 422 = _____

Answers: (a) 299 (b) 688 (c) 398 (d) 499 (e) 779 (f) 999 (g) 695 (h) 946 (i) 699 (j) 459 (k) 679
(l) 996.

If you want more practice, there are further examples at the end of the chapter.

You may have noticed that when you added each column, the answer was no more than 9. That was deliberate so that you could gain confidence before having to carry over a group of 10 to the next column. Let's look at how this is done. You only have to learn one rule and then apply it to as many columns as needed.

As you have already seen, our counting system uses **base 10**. All that you need to remember is that when the number is one greater than 9, that is 10, then you put 1 in the next column to the left.

Just remember that when you have 10 lots of 1 you write 10, for 10 lots of 10 you write 100 and when there are 10 lots of 100 you write 1000. When there are 10 lots of 1000, then it is written as 10 000 (ten thousand). The next step is hundreds of thousands and then 10 lots of 100 000 is a million, which is written as 1 000 000.

In these numbers, the zeros are crucial as they indicate the place value of the 1. They do not have any value in themselves but are **place holders**, keeping the 1 in the correct position. In scientific notation, there are no commas between the numbers but a gap is left between each group of three numbers, as here, starting from the right.

> **LOOK OUT**
>
> When dealing with patients' prescriptions, decimal points are often used when writing the dose. If commas are used, then they can be easily confused with a decimal point, which can result in a drug error.

> **KEY POINT**
>
> ● Numbers must be aligned under each other to ensure that they are not added incorrectly.

Carrying over a group of 10 to the next column

You have probably skipped through the chapter so far, which is the idea of the exercise. Don't hang around reading every bit if you are confident that you understand the rule and how to use it. Understanding is important, otherwise you will not be able to complete more complicated sums. Most problems arise because individuals have tried to remember the rule without knowing the underlying reason.

Now let's look at the rule of 10 again. The following calculations will test your understanding of addition of numbers that need you to carry one or more groups of 10 to the next column on the left.

```
        H  T  U
add +   2  7  6
        3  5  6
        ───────
        6  3  2
        1  1
```

As in the previous examples of adding hundreds, tens and units together, you must start from the units column on the right.

First the units column: $6 + 6 = 12$. Remember that this means one lot of 10 and two units over. It is useful to put the one 10 under the tens column, because you need to add it to the other tens.

You now have $7 + 5$ and the 1 that was carried over from the units column: $7 + 5 + 1 = 13$ (one lot of 100 and three lots of 10). Again there is one lot to be carried over, but this time it is 100, to go to the hundreds column.

Adding the hundreds column, 2 + 3 and the 1 carried over from the tens column: 2 + 3 + 1 = 6.

The answer to the sum is: 276 + 356 = 632.

This may seem a long-winded explanation, but if you understand the principles, then you can tackle any sum, no matter how many numbers have to be added together.

One more example:

```
        H  T  U
add +   4  7  7
        1  3  9
        3  2  5
        9  4  1
        1  2
```

In this case, the units column added up to 21, so there were two lots of 10 to be carried over to the tens column. What happens if there are more than 10 lots in the hundreds column? Another column has to be added for 'thousands'. You can set out the sum labelled **Th** (to distinguish it from **T** for tens) and put the thousands in that column. Another column to the left of that would be for tens of thousands (**TTh**) and then (**HTh**) hundreds of thousands and then a million (**M**).

In reality, when you are confident about what you are doing, there is no need to label the columns as long as the numbers are correctly aligned under each other. You should be able to do the smaller numbers without writing them down.

TIME TO TRY

(a) 237 + 98 = _____

(b) 173 + 348 = _____

(c) 532 + 389 = _____

(d) 196 + 144 = _____

(e) 372 + 88 = _____

(f) 83 + 594 = _____

(g) 456 + 127 + 197 = _____

(h) 43 + 547 + 18 = _____

(i) 183 + 24 + 519 = _____

(j) 92 + 314 + 675 = _____

(k) 739 + 33 + 92 = _____

(l) 821 + 67 + 814 = _____

Answers: (a) 335 (b) 521 (c) 921 (d) 340 (e) 460 (f) 677 (g) 780 (h) 608 (i) 726 (j) 1081 (k) 864 (l) 1702.

If you had some errors, check that you followed the rules. Make sure that you:

1. Aligned the numbers under each other before adding them together.

2. Carried over the tens and hundreds.

There are further examples at the end of the chapter if you need more practice.

APPLYING THE THEORY

You need to keep a record of the number of people that attend the outpatient department during the course of a week. The numbers for each day are as follows: Monday, 183; Tuesday, 215; Wednesday, 264; Thursday, 192; Friday, 117.

What is the total number of patients for the week?

Answer: 971 patients.

Addition is only one of the four basic operations of arithmetic but now you should be confident that you can cope with any whole numbers that need to be added together.

1.2 SUBTRACTION

YOUR STARTING POINT FOR SUBTRACTION

Without using a calculator, write down the answers to the following questions.

(a) 5 − 4 = _____   (b) 7 − 3 = _____

(c) 12 − 8 = _____   (d) 17 − 13 = _____

(e) 25 − 15 = _____   (f) 47 − 33 = _____

(g) 127 − 111 = _____   (h) 246 − 137 = _____

(i) 323 − 195 = _____   (j) 1376 − 1125 = _____

(k) 3322 − 1782 = _____   (l) 2571 − 1684 = _____

Answers: (a) 1 (b) 4 (c) 4 (d) 4 (e) 10 (f) 14 (g) 16 (h) 109 (i) 128 (j) 251 (k) 1540 (l) 887.

If you had these all correct, skip through to Section 1.3 – Multiplication.

Subtraction means taking one number away from another. The second number is taken from the first. The answer is what is left over.

You can use the number line to help you to become confident about taking away:

<u>0 1 2 3 4 5 6 7 8 9 10 11 12 13 14 15 16 17 18 19 20</u>

Use the number line to work out this sum: 10 − 4. Start at 10 and count back 4, to the left. You are taking 4 away from 10. This will give you the answer 6. You can check that you are right by adding the number you took away to your answer. It should give you the first number of the sum: 10 − 4 = 6. (Check: 6 + 4 = 10.)

Maybe you are now starting to see the relationship between addition and subtraction?

TIME TO TRY

(a) 7 − 3 = _____　　(b) 9 − 4 = _____　　(c) 6 − 2 = _____

(d) 8 − 3 = _____　　(e) 3 − 2 = _____　　(f) 4 − 1 = _____

(g) 9 − 6 = _____　　(h) 1 − 0 = _____　　(i) 16 − 9 = _____

(j) 18 − 12 = _____　　(k) 20 − 7 = _____　　(l) 13 − 7 = _____

Answers: (a) 4 (b) 5 (c) 4 (d) 5 (e) 1 (f) 3 (g) 3 (h) 1 (i) 7 (j) 6 (k) 13 (l) 6.

More examples are at the end of the chapter if you need more practice.

You can subtract simple numbers in your head but as they get bigger, you might find it helpful to use one of the following methods:

1. Partitioning, or breaking up the numbers and subtracting them in turn:

$$43 − 36 \text{ is the same as } 43 − 30 − 6$$
$$43 − 30 = 13$$
$$13 − 6 − 17$$
$$43 − 36 = 17$$

2. Use near numbers and adjust:

$$43 − 19 = 43 − 20 + 1 = 23 + 1 = 24$$

Here you use a number that is near the number in the sum but is easier to use, which in this case is 20 instead of 19. You have to take this into account in your final answer, so if you have taken off one more than you needed, then you have to add it onto your answer.

3. Counting on. When you worked out the number bonds for 10, 20 and 100, you used the method that was called counting on. You can also use this way to get the answer to subtraction problems.

To work out 53 − 36, count on from 36 to 53:

Count on from 36 to 40 to get 4
Count on from 40 to 50 to get 10
Count on from 50 to 53 to get 3
4 + 10 + 3 = 17

$$36 \xrightarrow{} 40 \xrightarrow{} 50 \xrightarrow{} 53$$
$$\ \ 4 \qquad\quad 10 \qquad\quad 3$$

You may find your own way of making things easier; it doesn't matter which method you use as long as you get the right answer and understand how you got there.

Subtraction is the opposite of addition, so you can check you are right by adding your answer to the number which was subtracted.

To check that $53 - 36 = 17$, add the 17 and the 36 and you should get 53.

If the numbers are too large or too difficult to subtract in your head, you can write them down in columns, as you did with addition; always start subtracting with the units.

$$
\begin{array}{ccc}
\text{H} & \text{T} & \text{U} \\
6 & 5 & 8 \\
\hline
2 & 2 & 3 \\
\hline
4 & 3 & 5 \\
\end{array}
$$

subtract −

Borrowing

Sometimes one of the columns has a smaller number on top, and so the number on top borrows from the number to its left. You will have to carry out a couple more steps to get your answer.

$$
\begin{array}{ccc}
\text{H} & \text{T} & \text{U} \\
6 & {}^{4}5 & {}^{1}8 \\
\hline
2 & 2 & 9 \\
\hline
4 & 2 & 9 \\
\end{array}
$$

subtract −

In the units column of this example the top number is 8 and you are asked to subtract 9. The solution is to '**borrow**' a 10 from the tens column, change it to 10 units and add it in the units column. Now you are left with 4 in the tens column and 18 in the units. It is now possible to take 9 away from 18, leaving 9 units.

This method can be used whether the larger number involved is in the units, tens, hundreds, thousands or any other column.

It's a good idea to estimate a rough answer first and always check your actual answer. Thus 658 is nearly 660 and 229 is nearly 230, so an estimate of your answer is $660 - 230 = 430$. (You can do it in your head.) It is even more important to have a rough estimate of the expected answer when you are using a calculator.

Borrowing because of a zero

This is the same because, if one of the columns has a smaller number on top, you borrow from the number to its left.

$$
\begin{array}{ccc}
\text{H} & \text{T} & \text{U} \\
{}^{5}6 & {}^{1}0 & 8 \\
\hline
2 & 2 & 7 \\
\hline
3 & 8 & 1 \\
\end{array}
$$

subtract −

When working out the tens in this sum, because 0 is less than 2, you have to borrow 10 from the hundreds column. So 0 becomes 10. In the hundreds column you now have 5 lots of hundreds.

KEY POINT

● When the number in the top row of the subtraction sum is smaller than the one in the bottom row, then you need to borrow one from the next column on the left.

TIME TO TRY

(a) 29 − 18 = _____

(b) 35 − 21 = _____

(c) 47 − 29 = _____

(d) 77 − 48 = _____

(e) 93 − 44 = _____

(f) 84 − 37 = _____

(g) 187 − 75 = _____

(h) 124 − 105 = _____

(i) 278 − 166 = _____

(j) 536 − 218 = _____

(k) 409 − 217 = _____

(l) 627 − 348 = _____

Answers: (a) 11 (b) 14 (c) 18 (d) 29 (e) 49 (f) 47 (g) 112 (h) 19 (i) 112 (j) 318 (k) 192 (l) 279.

More examples are at the end of the chapter.

APPLYING THE THEORY

Many patients need to have the amount of fluid that they drink and the volume of urine passed carefully measured. Normally the difference between intake and output is less than 200 millilitres.

Remember that 'difference' is a word indicating subtraction. If a patient's total intake is 1995 millilitres and the urinary output measures as 1875 then you need to subtract:

$$1955 - 1875 = 80$$

The difference between intake and output is 80 millilitres, which is what would be expected under normal circumstances.

 Monitoring fluid balance is important so that the correct treatment is given. There will be more details about fluid balance monitoring in Chapter 8.

Negative numbers

We write negative numbers like this:

negative 2 is the same as ⁻2

The raised dash is the negative sign. It is usually written slightly shorter and a little higher up than a normal minus sign, but on the Internet and in newspapers you will see it written using a minus sign.

Sometimes negative numbers are called *minus* numbers. Be careful that you don't confuse these with subtraction.

The time when you are most likely to come across **negative numbers** is in the winter weather forecast. If the temperature is below 0°C then it is very cold and as the minus number increases, so the temperature gets colder: minus 5 (−5) degrees centigrade is colder than −2°C. This is the opposite of **positive numbers**, which indicate that the weather is getting warmer as the number increases.

Look at the number line below. Negative numbers are always written to the left of the zero on graphs and number lines and positive ones to the right.

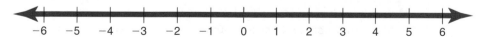

Another instance may be your bank balance at the end of the month! If you owe £3, you are minus three pounds. If someone else owes £5, they have an even greater negative state than you. If you are then given £2, then your −£3 is reduced to −£1. Find −3 on the number line and add 2; that is, move to the right. You will find that you are at −1. If you are then given a further £5, you will then have a positive balance of £4.

APPLYING THE THEORY

If a patient is given drugs to make them pass more urine, you would expect that when you calculate the difference between the amount of fluid in and fluid out, they would have less fluid intake than output. We say that they have a negative fluid balance. For example,

total intake 1360 millilitres   total output 1950 millilitres

You then need to find out the difference between the two numbers. Take the smaller number away from the larger number: 1950 − 1360 = 590.

You can see that the body has lost more fluid than was retained. In this case 590 millilitres more has been lost. This is a negative balance: the body has ⁻590 millilitres less than the previous 24 hours.

1.3 MULTIPLICATION

YOUR STARTING POINT FOR MULTIPLICATION

Without using a calculator, write down the answers to the following questions.

(a) 4 × 5 = _____   (b) 3 × 7 = _____

(c) 8 × 8 = _____   (d) 9 × 7 = _____

(e) 5 × 5 = _____   (f) 6 × 3 = _____

(g) 12 × 2 = _____   (h) 10 × 7 = _____

(i) 15 × 6 = _____   (j) 39 × 23 = _____

(k) 115 × 25 = _____   (l) 245 × 100 = _____

Answers: (a) 20 (b) 21 (c) 64 (d) 63 (e) 25 (f) 18 (g) 24 (h) 70 (i) 90 (j) 897 (k) 2875 (l) 24 500.

If you had all these correct, you can move on to Section 1.4 – Division.

Multiplication is much easier if you know your times tables. You can use **Table 1.3** to help you brush up. Choose a number in the left-hand column and one from the top row, and where the column and row meet in the table is the answer to the multiplication, e.g. 6 × 8 = 48. You will also see that if you take 8 in the left-hand column and 6 in the top row, you will get the same answer.

Remember that if you multiply any number by 1, the number doesn't change, but if it is multiplied by 0 your answer is zero. Not logical? If you have no money and you multiply it by 7 you still have no money!

If you look at the table, you will see in the ×10 column that when a number is multiplied by 10, the answer is the number followed by 0, e.g. 5 × 10 = 50, 9 × 10 = 90.

This pattern is true of any number multiplied by 10. What is 273 × 10?

Answer: 2730.

When a number is multiplied by 100, the figures move two places to the left and two zeros are added to the spaces, e.g. 2 × 100 = 200, 345 × 100 = 34 500.

Table 1.3 Multiplication using a grid

×	0	1	2	3	4	5	6	7	8	9	10
0	0	0	0	0	0	0	0	0	0	0	0
1	0	1	2	3	4	5	6	7	8	9	10
2	0	2	4	6	8	10	12	14	16	18	20
3	0	3	6	9	12	15	18	21	24	27	30
4	0	4	8	12	16	20	24	28	32	36	40
5	0	5	10	15	20	25	30	35	40	45	50
6	0	6	12	18	24	30	36	42	48	54	60
7	0	7	14	21	28	35	42	49	56	63	70
8	0	8	16	24	32	40	48	56	64	72	80
9	0	9	18	27	36	45	54	63	72	81	90
10	0	10	20	30	40	50	60	70	80	90	100

APPLYING THE THEORY

You will often have to multiply by 10, 100 and 1000 when converting units for calculating drug doses, so it is important that you can do it quickly and accurately. You will learn more about changing units in a later chapter.

If you are multiplying numbers you need to decide whether to do the calculation in your head or write it down.

When you multiply, remember that you will expect the number of your answer to be bigger than those that you multiplied together.

Multiplication is a quick way of doing addition. If you find that odd, think about this straightforward example: $5 \times 6 = 30$. You may have learned the five times table and know the answer without any trouble and may not have thought about what it really meant. We can think of 5×6 as five lots of six. If you write down five sixes in a column and make an addition sum:

```
        T   U
            6
            6
    +       6
            6
            6
        ───────
        3   0
```

Similarly 25×3 is 25 lots of three. It is tedious writing 3 down 25 times and adding them, but in multiplication it does not matter which number is multiplied by which. So it is just as valid to write 3 lots of 25:

```
        T   U
        2   5
        2   5
        2   5
        ───────
        7   5
        1
```

Place value again

In the number 293, 2 means two hundreds, 9 means nine tens and 3 means three units:

```
    H   T   U
    2   0   0  ───────▶  two hundreds
        9   0  ───────▶  nine tens
            3  ───────▶  three units
    ─────────────
    2   9   3
```

You can use this method of breaking up a large number to simplify the multiplication of big numbers. If the sum is 293×6, then one way of doing the sum is to multiply each row by 6:

$$200 \times 6 = 1200$$
$$90 \times 6 = 540$$
$$3 \times 6 = 18$$

The numbers are then added together to get the answer: $1200 + 540 + 18 = 1758$.

Traditional method of multiplication

You may be more familiar with the following way of multiplication. We use the same sum as before, 293×6, using this method.

First we set out the sum in the following way:

```
Th  H  T  U
     2  9  3
×           6
_____
_____
```

Now we multiply the number in each column by 6, starting with the units:

(a) $6 \times 3 = 18$. Put 8 in the units column and carry 1 to the tens.

(b) $6 \times 9 = 54$. Add the 1 carried over to make 55.

(c) One 5 goes in the tens column and 5 is carried over to the hundreds column.

(d) $6 \times 2 = 12$. Add the 5 carried over to make 17.

(e) The 7 is put in the hundreds column and the one in the thousands.

So $293 \times 6 = 1758$.

```
Th  H  T  U
     2  9  3
×           6
_____
 1   7  5  8
 1   5  1
```

TIME TO TRY

Use whichever method you prefer for the following or experiment to see which you find easier.

(a) $15 \times 5 = $ _____   (b) $18 \times 0 = $ _____   (c) $37 \times 9 = $ _____

(d) $87 \times 4 = $ _____   (e) $2 \times 385 = $ _____   (f) $643 \times 3 = $ _____

(g) $948 \times 8 = $ _____   (h) $7 \times 587 = $ _____   (i) $467 \times 1 = $ _____

(j) $2791 \times 6 = $ _____ (k) $3755 \times 9 = $ _____   (l) $1768 \times 7 = $ _____

Answers: (a) 75 (b) 0 (c) 333 (d) 348 (e) 770 (f) 1929 (g) 7584 (h) 4109 (i) 467 (j) 16746 (k) 33 795 (l) 12 376.

More examples, if you need them, are at the end of the chapter.

Even larger numbers

If you have a sum where the numbers that you have to multiply are both two figures or more, each figure is multiplied separately. It is even more important to understand place value because the number that you are multiplying by is broken up.

EXAMPLE

Calculate 376 × 35. Multiplying by 35 is the same as multiplying by 30 and then by 5.
    First multiply 376 by the unit 5:

(a) 5 × 6 = 30. Put the 0 in the units column and carry 3 to the tens.

(b) 5 × 7 = 35. Add the 3 carried over, which makes 38.
    8 goes in the tens column and the 3 is carried over to the hundreds column.

(c) 5 × 3 = 15. Add the 3 carried over from the tens column, which makes 18.
    8 goes in the hundreds column and 1 in the thousands.

This makes a total of 1880.

    Next multiply 376 by the tens digit 3. When multiplying by tens you must remember to add the zero first in the units column because you are really multiplying by 30. (Remember from Table 1.2 that any number multiplied by 10 has a zero added at the end.)

(a) 3 × 6 = 18. Put the 8 in the tens column and carry 1 to the hundreds.

(b) 3 × 7 = 21. Add the 1 carried over from the tens column, which makes 22.
    2 goes in the hundreds column and the other 2 is carried over to the thousands column.

(c) 3 × 3 = 9. Add the 2 carried over from the hundreds column, which makes 11.
    1 goes in the thousands column and the other one in the tens of thousands.

This makes a total of 11 280.

    To find the answer to the original question, 376 × 35, we need to add the two sums together: 1880 + 11 280 = 13 160.

$$
\begin{array}{rccccc}
 & \text{TTh} & \text{Th} & \text{H} & \text{T} & \text{U} \\
 & & & 3 & 7 & 6 \\
\times & & & & 3 & 5 \\
\hline
 & & 1 & 8_3 & 8_3 & 0 \\
 & 1 & 1_2 & 2_1 & 8 & 0 \quad \text{add} \\
\hline
 & 1 & 3_1 & 1_1 & 6 & 0 \\
\hline
\end{array}
$$

APPLYING THE THEORY

Some drug dosages are calculated according to the patient's weight, so it may be necessary for you to multiply the dose per kilogram by the patient's weight in kilograms.

If a patient weighs 64 kg and they have to be given 15 mg for each kilogram of their body weight, in order to find out how much of the drug that they need the amount of drug per kilogram has to be multiplied by the number of kilograms, so 15×64 gives the number of milligrams to be given. This is a total of 960 mg.

```
        H  T  U
           6  4
     ×     1  5
        3  2₂ 0
        6  4  0    add
        9  6  0
```

TIME TO TRY

(a) $478 \times 48 =$ _____

(b) $396 \times 87 =$ _____

(c) $727 \times 57 =$ _____

(d) $592 \times 34 =$ _____

(e) $653 \times 64 =$ _____

(f) $295 \times 76 =$ _____

(g) $589 \times 53 =$ _____

(h) $178 \times 96 =$ _____

(i) $237 \times 85 =$ _____

(j) $344 \times 46 =$ _____

(k) $876 \times 35 =$ _____

(l) $144 \times 69 =$ _____

Answers: (a) 22 944 (b) 34 452 (c) 41 439 (d) 20 128 (e) 41 792 (f) 22 420 (g) 31 217 (h) 17 088 (i) 20 145 (j) 15 824 (k) 30 660 (l) 9936.

Further questions are at the end of the chapter.

1.4 DIVISION

YOUR STARTING POINT FOR DIVISION

(a) $10 \div 5 =$ _____

(b) $21 \div 7 =$ _____

(c) $64 \div 8 =$ _____

(d) $504 \div 9 =$ _____

(e) $105 \div 5 =$ _____

(f) $36 \div 3 =$ _____

(g) $345 \div 15 =$ _____

(h) $121 \div 11 =$ _____

(i) $7125 \div 57 =$ _____

(j) $425 \div 17 =$ _____

(k) $125 \div 25 =$ _____

(l) $812 \div 14 =$ _____

Answers: (a) 2 (b) 3 (c) 8 (d) 56 (e) 21 (f) 12 (g) 23 (h) 11 (i) 125 (j) 25 (k) 5 (l) 58.

If you had all these correct, go to Section 1.5.

Division is really repeated subtraction, and is the opposite of multiplication.

Sharing is a form of division. Say you have a packet of biscuits that has to be shared between five people. You can give a biscuit to each person and share them around until there are no more left in the packet. You find that they have four biscuits each. If five people have four biscuits each and there are none left, the packet must have contained $5 \times 4 = 20$ biscuits.

If you had counted the biscuits before you shared them then you could have divided the number of biscuits by the number of people who were sharing them: $20 \div 5 = 4$. Division problems must be done from left to right. Reading out aloud 'twenty divided by five' helps you to identify the number that is to be divided.

As you saw in Table 1.1, there are several ways of indicating that numbers have to be divided. The number to be divided is called the **dividend** and the number which divides is called the **divisor**. In the examples below, 20 is the dividend and 5 the divisor. The answer is called the **quotient**, which in this case is 4. These are all ways of setting out the same division.

$$20 \div 5 \qquad \frac{20}{5} \qquad 5\overline{)20} \qquad 20/5 \qquad 5\underline{)\ 20}$$

Again you should be able to do these without using a calculator.

You can check your answer to a division by multiplying the answer by the divisor, which will give you the number that was the dividend:

$$72 \div 8 = 9 \qquad 9 \times 8 = 72$$

There are a number of ways that you can make division easier to carry out when you are not using a calculator.

You can break up the number being divided to make it easier to handle. If you want to divide $52 \div 4$, 52 can be split into 40 and 12, both of which can be divided by 4:

$$40 \div 4 = 10 \quad \text{and} \quad 12 \div 4 = 3$$

Add the two answers together: $10 + 3 = 13$. So $52 \div 4 = 13$.

Another way of making life easier is to split the number that is the divisor into its factors (smaller numbers which, when multiplied, make up the divisor). If you want to divide $525 \div 15$, 15 can be split into the factors $5 \times 3 = 15$. Then 525 can be divided first by 5 and the answer divided by 3. This is easier than dividing by 15.

$$525 \div 5 = 105 \quad \text{and} \quad 105 \div 3 = 35$$

So $525 \div 15 = 35$.

TIME TO TRY

(a) $27 \div 9 =$ _____

(b) $72 \div 6 =$ _____

(c) $15 \div 5 =$ _____

(d) $45 \div 5 =$ _____

(e) $189 \div 3 =$ _____

(f) $81 \div 9 =$ _____

(g) $120 \div 8 =$ _____

(h) $150 \div 6 =$ _____

(i) $126 \div 6 =$ _____

(j) $63 \div 3 =$ _____

(k) $35 \div 7 =$ _____

(l) $28 \div 4 =$ _____

Answers: (a) 3 (b) 12 (c) 3 (d) 9 (e) 63 (f) 9 (g) 15 (h) 25 (i) 21 (j) 21 (k) 5 (l) 7.

There are more examples at the end of the chapter.

Long division

The sum $36\,265 \div 5$ can be set out as below to make it easier to handle larger numbers. As long as you know your five times table this is not a problem.

$$\begin{array}{r} 7\ 2\ 5\ 3 \\ \hline 5)\overline{3\ ^36\ ^12\ ^26\ ^15} \end{array}$$

If you take this in steps, you will see that this is a straightforward way of doing this type of division. Put each number of the answer above the appropriate column of the dividend.

(a) 5 into 3 won't go, so carry 3 over to the 6.

(b) 5 into 36: 5 × **7** = 35, the remainder of 1 to be carried over to the 2.

(c) 5 into 12: 5 × **2** = 10, the remainder of 2 to be carried over to the 6.

(d) 5 into 26: 5 × **5** = 25, the remainder of 1 to be carried over to the 5.

(e) 5 into 15: 5 × **3** = 15, no remainder.

The answer is 7253.

   Long division involving divisors above 10, with the exception of 100, 1000 and 1 000 000, will be discussed later. You will be glad to know that these will be done using a calculator!

TIME TO TRY

(a) $20 \div 5 =$ _____

(b) $63 \div 7 =$ _____

(c) $56 \div 8 =$ _____

(d) $81 \div 9 =$ _____

(e) $105 \div 5 =$ _____

(f) $93 \div 3 =$ _____

(g) $312 \div 6 =$ _____

(h) $132 \div 12 =$ _____

(i) $7125 \div 5 =$ _____

(j) $1968 \div 3 =$ _____

(k) $343 \div 7 =$ _____

(l) $4336 \div 8 =$ _____

Answers: (a) 4 (b) 9 (c) 7 (d) 9 (e) 21 (f) 31 (g) 52 (h) 11 (i) 1425 (j) 656 (k) 49 (l) 542.

There are more examples at the end of the chapter.

APPLYING THE THEORY

Injections of drugs are packaged in glass containers, and often a patient is prescribed a dose that is only part of the amount in the container. This means that you will have to divide the volume in the container to get the right dose. You need to be able to work out the sum and get it right. A calculator should not be relied solely upon for the answer; you need to know what answer to expect.

1.5 EXPONENTS AND SCIENTIFIC NOTATION

You may have heard the expression two squared or two to the power of two. It is written as 2^2. The small number is called an **exponent** or index (plural indices). It means $2 \times 2 = 4$. Similarly $2^4 = 2 \times 2 \times 2 \times 2 = 16$.

In laboratory reports very large and very small numbers are written using exponents in a form called scientific notation. When there is a large number of zeros, it can be confusing to read and one could be added or missed when written.

$$10 \times 10 = 100 = 10^2 \qquad 10 \times 10 \times 10 = 1000 = 10^3$$

$$10 \times 10 \times 10 \times 10 \times 10 \times 10 = 1\,000\,000 = 10^6$$

It is easy to multiply and divide numbers with **indices**. The index tells you how many times the number is multiplied by itself.

$$\text{Multiply} \quad 100 \times 100 = 10^2 \times 10^2$$

$$10\,000 = 10^4$$

As you can see, adding the indices gives you the answer very quickly.

Similarly, you can divide numbers with exponents by subtracting the indices.

$$\text{Divide} \quad 2^6 \div 2^3$$

$$2 \times 2 \times 2 \times 2 \times 2 \times 2 = 64 \div 2 \times 2 \times 2 = 8$$

$$64 \div 8 = 8$$

If you subtract the indices

$$2^6 \div 2^3 = 2^3 = 2 \times 2 \times 2 = 8$$

This is much easier than writing out the sum in full. It eliminates the danger of missing or adding a 2.

You can only add and subtract indices if the big numbers are the same.

There will be more about exponents in later chapters.

KEY POINTS

- Exponents are a convenient way of expressing large numbers.
- Indices can be added if the numbers are to be multiplied or subtracted if the numbers are divided.

APPLYING THE THEORY

Look at the blood reports that come from the laboratory. You will see that a red blood cell count is reported as the number of cells contained in 1 litre of blood. A normal count will be reported as 5×10^{12}/L, which if written out in full would be 5 000 000 000 000 cells per litre.

Using a calculator

At last you can get out your calculator! It is a useful tool but you must not rely on it. You need to check your answer by having done an estimate of the answer. You may not always have a calculator but you do have your head!

Figure 1.1 shows a basic calculator. You don't need a more complicated one but the important thing is that you read the instruction book! It is quite useful if you have a calculator that shows the sum as you put in the figures, because you can check for errors on the way.

First check that the display panel is clear by pressing the ON/C button.

Addition

Adding is straightforward – you just enter the numbers as they come in the sum, e.g. 29 + 48.

What is your rough estimate?

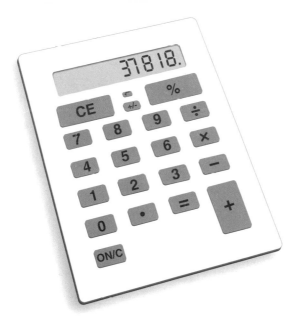

Figure 1.1 Pocket calculator

Now 29 is nearly 30 and 48 is nearly 50, so you would expect your answer to be nearly 80. In fact, with all the practice you have had you don't really need to use the calculator!

Now try putting the sum into the calculator:

Press 2, then 9, then + and then press 4, then 8, then =

The answer, 77, will appear in the display panel.

Try these sums to see if they have been entered into the calculator correctly.

(a) 75 + 84 = 159   (b) 65 + 76 = 131   (c) 34 + 87 = 121

(d) 123 + 124 = 247   (e) 4556 + 8679 = 13225

Sums (b) and (e) both have errors. It is easy to push the wrong button, especially if you have a calculator with small buttons. Many of the free ones fall into this category, so you would do well to look that particular gift horse in the mouth!

Subtraction

Subtraction is carried out in a similar way, entering the numbers as they are written in the sum. Try it on your calculator: say, 87 − 39. Make sure that you have cancelled all your previous calculations before you do by pressing the ON/C key.

The answer is 48.

Multiplication

On some calculators the multiplication symbol is × but on others it is * so check the machine that you are using.

It does not matter which number you put in first but it is good practice to go from the left as you will have to do this later. Try this one: 49 × 25.

Answer: 1225.

Division

The symbol for division varies between calculators. On some, it is a / and on others it is a ÷ sign.

It *does* matter in which order you input the figures. Say the sum aloud if you need to remind yourself which number is the dividend and which the divisor. The dividend has to be entered first. Try this one: 9045 ÷ 15.

Answer: 603.

And finally!

Now you have learned the four basic operations of arithmetic there is one more set of rules for dealing with calculations that involve more than one type of operation. You need to know about **BODMAS**!

Look at the following sum: $4 + 6 \times 3$.

If you calculate $4 + 6$ first you then have $10 \times 3 = 30$
If you calculate 6×3 first you then have $4 + 18 = 22$
Two different answers; which one is right?

This is where BODMAS comes in. It is an acronym to tell you in which order the calculation must be done:

B brackets, e.g. $(7 + 9)$, $(7 - 9)$, $(9 \div 3)$

O other operations, anything that is not one of the four basic operations, e.g. 5^3

D division, e.g. $10 \div 2$

M multiplication, e.g. 4×8

A addition, e.g. $8 + 3$

S subtraction, e.g. $9 - 4$

You might like to make up a phrase to help you remember the order, for example:

Big **O**rang-utans **D**oze **M**oodily **A**fter **S**upper

Try this one:

$$2 + 3 \times 5 - 4$$

You should have multiplied 3×5 first.
Then the sum is

$$2 + 15 - 4 = 13$$

Now try this one

$$4 \times (9 - 4)$$

Although multiplication is done before subtraction, because the subtraction part of the question is in brackets, it gets done first.

Answer: 20, i.e. $4 \times (9 - 4) = 4 \times 5 = 20$.

Try these, using the BODMAS rules.

(a) $3 \times 6 + 7 =$ _____

(b) $32 \div (18 - 10) =$ _____

(c) $(5 + 4) \times (7 - 2) =$ _____

(d) $(5 + 4) \times 7 - 2 =$ _____

(e) $8^2 - 6 \times 6 =$ _____

(f) $15 + 3 \times (4 - 2) =$ _____

Answers: (a) 25 (b) 4 (c) 45 (d) 61 (e) 28 (f) 21.

If you remembered the rule then these should have been no trouble! If not, here is how they are worked:

(a) First multiply $3 \times 6 = 18$ then add $7 = 25$.

(b) First subtract 10 from $18 = 8$ then divide 32 by $8 = 4$.

(c) Do the brackets first $5 + 4 = 9$ then subtract 2 from $7 = 5$. Finally multiply $5 \times 9 = 45$.

(d) Brackets first $5 + 4 = 9$. Now multiply $9 \times 7 = 63$ then subtract $2 = 61$.

(e) Exponent first $8^2 = 8 \times 8 = 64$. Multiply $6 \times 6 = 36$, then subtract 36 from $64 = 28$.

(f) Brackets first $4 - 2 = 2$. Now multiply $3 \times 2 = 6$, then add $15 + 6 = 21$.

There will be more use of BODMAS later in calculations of physiological parameters.

RUNNING WORDS

addition	dividend	near number	place value
base 10	division	negative number	positive number
BODMAS	divisor	number bond	quotient
borrowing	exponent	numeral	subtraction
carrying over	indices	partitioning	
counting on	multiplication	place holder	

Answers to the following questions can be found at the end of the book.

What did you learn?

Answer the following questions without using a calculator.

(a) $25 + 47 =$ _____

(b) $291 \div 3 =$ _____

(c) $563 \times 8 =$ _____

(d) $58 - 43 =$ _____

(e) $847 + 362 + 178 =$ _____

(f) $874 \times 46 =$ _____

(g) $2275 \div 7 =$ _____

(h) $5736 - 1845 =$ _____

(i) $4^3 =$ _____

(j) $10^5 \times 10^4 =$ _____

(k) $3 \times 5 + 6 - 2 =$ _____

(l) $4 \times (8 - 2) + 3 =$ _____

More 'Time to Try' examples

Number bonds 1 to 100, page 7

(a) 70 + _____ = 100   (b) 25 + _____ = 100   (c) 47 + _____ = 100

(d) 88 + _____ = 100   (e) 13 + _____ = 100   (f) 51 + _____ = 100

(g) 19 + _____ = 100   (h) 62 + _____ = 100   (i) 46 + _____ = 100

(j) 33 + _____ = 100   (k) 73 + _____ = 100   (l) 57 + _____ = 100

Addition, page 8

(a) 20 + 130 + 19 = _____   (b) 524 + 121 + 153 = _____

(c) 104 + 201 + 93 = _____   (d) 23 + 310 + 46 = _____

(e) 102 + 434 + 63 = _____   (f) 701 + 162 + 132 = _____

(g) 530 + 117 + 241 = _____   (h) 214 + 422 + 362 = _____

(i) 242 + 11 + 43 = _____   (j) 211 + 322 + 163 = _____

(k) 431 + 131 + 332 = _____   (l) 621 + 35 + 143 = _____

Addition – carrying over, page 10

(a) 338 + 68 = _____   (b) 184 + 398 = _____

(c) 325 + 487 = _____   (d) 495 + 686 = _____

(e) 483 + 77 = _____   (f) 63 + 678 = _____

(g) 835 + 236 + 283 = _____   (h) 53 + 583 + 19 = _____

(i) 346 + 42 + 453 = _____   (j) 739 + 27 + 521 = _____

(k) 153 + 356 + 33 = _____   (l) 617 + 546 + 63 = _____

Subtraction, page 12

(a) 9 − 5 = _____   (b) 10 − 5 = _____

(c) 8 − 4 = _____   (d) 7 − 2 = _____

(e) 9 − 2 = _____   (f) 7 − 4 = _____

(g) 10 − 7 = _____   (h) 3 − 0 = _____

(i) 14 − 9 = _____   (j) 14 − 8 = _____

(k) 20 − 6 = _____   (l) 18 − 12 = _____

Subtraction with borrowing, page 14

(a) 43 − 19 = _____   (b) 65 − 26 = _____

(c) 34 − 18 = _____   (d) 84 − 48 = _____

(e) 103 − 44 = _____   (f) 93 − 37 = _____

(g) 152 − 65 = _____   (h) 144 − 106 = _____

(i) 369 − 176 = _____   (j) 836 − 279 = _____

(k) 509 − 229 = _____   (l) 738 − 398 = _____

Multiplication, page 18

(a) 14 × 5 = _____   (b) 15 × 0 = _____

(c) 39 × 9 = _____   (d) 77 × 4 = _____

(e) 2 × 194 = _____   (f) 724 × 3 = _____

(g) 582 × 8 = _____   (h) 7 × 182 = _____

(i) 599 × 1 = _____   (j) 2644 × 6 = _____

(k) 3788 × 9 = _____   (l) 1245 × 7 = _____

Multiplication, page 20

(a) 578 × 58 = _____   (b) 496 × 94 = _____

(c) 827 × 68 = _____   (d) 492 × 24 = _____

(e) 343 × 46 = _____   (f) 235 × 83 = _____

(g) 136 × 53 = _____   (h) 152 × 47 = _____

(i) 293 × 74 = _____   (j) 473 × 62 = _____

(k) 215 × 93 = _____   (l) 579 × 37 = _____

Division, page 21-22

(a) 40 ÷ 5 = _____   (b) 63 ÷ 3 = _____

(c) 56 ÷ 7 = _____   (d) 108 ÷ 9 = _____

(e) 210 ÷ 5 = _____   (f) 84 ÷ 3 = _____

(g) 132 ÷ 6 = _____   (h) 3138 ÷ 6 = _____

(i) 9675 ÷ 5 = _____   (j) 2142 ÷ 6 = _____

(k) 2478 ÷ 7 = _____   (l) 1480 ÷ 8 = _____

Web resources

BBC websites

http://www.bbc.co.uk/skillswise/numbers
This site is aimed at all family members so there are examples at all levels of ability and covering the topics dealt with in this chapter.

http://www.bbc.co.uk/schools/gcsebitesize/maths/
Primarily for preparation for GCSE from foundation to intermediate level, which is roughly the minimum standard you will need to reach.

http://www.bbc.co.uk/schools/ks2bitesize/
Key Stage 2 is a good level to aim at before the end of Chapter 4. You need to concentrate on the material covered in this chapter and move on to other topics as you progress through the book or when you feel ready.

Maths for fun

http://www.mathsisfun.com
Look at the multiplication and division sections. There are animations of the calculations, which may help you if you are better at learning visually. This is an American site so is not so useful later when you need to get to grips with the metric system.

http://www.easymaths.com
This site will convert you to thinking that maths can be fun as well as brushing up on the basic skills.

http://www.headstartinbiology.com
You will have to register for this site (it's free!). Gallery 1 is mainly geared towards maths and measurement used in healthcare.

Chapter 2

Decimals and other fractions

How to deal with the bits and pieces

When drugs come from the manufacturer they are in doses to suit most adult patients. However, many of your patients will be very young or very old and they need smaller doses. You may need to calculate the correct amount by taking part or a fraction of the standard dose, so you need to understand how to work out fractions.

When you have completed this chapter, you should be able to:

- Add, subtract, multiply and divide vulgar fractions.
- Add, subtract, multiply and divide decimal fractions.

In Chapter 1 you got to grips with the four basic operations of arithmetic using whole numbers. This chapter takes you a small step further in using the skills that you have already learned, so that you can tackle calculations that involve parts of a whole number, known as fractions.

2.1 ADDITION OF VULGAR FRACTIONS

YOUR STARTING POINT FOR ADDITION OF FRACTIONS

Without using a calculator, write down the answers to the following in their *simplest form:*

(a) 1/4 + 1/2 = _____   (b) 1/4 + 2/3 = _____

(c) 3/7 + 2/5 = _____   (d) 5/8 + 3/6 = _____

(e) 3/5 + 7/10 = _____   (f) 3/4 + 5/6 = _____

(g) $7\frac{1}{5} + 4\frac{1}{3}$ = _____   (h) $2\frac{1}{7} + 3\frac{3}{8}$ = _____

(i) $1\frac{2}{3} + 5\frac{5}{6}$ = _____

Answers: (a) 3/4 (b) 11/12 (c) $\frac{29}{35}$ (d) $1\frac{1}{8}$ (e) $1\frac{3}{10}$ (f) $1\frac{7}{12}$ (g) $11\frac{8}{15}$ (h) $5\frac{29}{56}$ (i) $7\frac{1}{2}$.

If you had all these correct, well done; now go to Section 2.2, the starting point for subtraction of fractions.

Vulgar fractions are written with one number over another, separated by a line. If you remember Table 1.1, this was one way of indicating that a number was divided by another.

You are probably very familiar with some vulgar fractions: for example, a half is written as 1/2, which also means one divided by two. Fractions can also be written as $\frac{1}{2}$ or 1/2.

The number below the line is called the **denominator** and tells you how many parts into which the whole has been split.

The number above the line is the **numerator** and tells you the number of parts of the whole number that are being used.

If you have an apple pie and it is cut into five equal pieces, then each piece is $\frac{1}{5}$ (one-fifth) of the whole pie (**Figure 2.1**).

If you, your brother and a friend each take a slice, then you will have two pieces left. This can be written as $\frac{2}{5}$ of the whole are left (**Figure 2.2**) and $\frac{3}{5}$ of the whole have been eaten. (There will be none left shortly, so do the calculation quickly.)

If you add the fraction representing the number of pieces left to the number of pieces eaten, you will get

$$\frac{2}{5} + \frac{3}{5} = \frac{5}{5} = 1$$

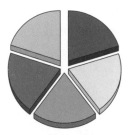

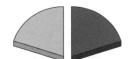

Figure 2.1 A pie cut into five equal pieces

Figure 2.2 Two fifths of the pie are left

If you say this aloud, you will hear that the sum says 'Two fifths plus three fifths'. The denominators of each fraction indicate the number of parts into which the whole has been divided. In this case they are the same, fifths, so these are not changed. If you add the numerators together then, again, you have 5 as the number on top.

Do you remember the meaning of the line between the two fives? It is another way of saying divide, so $5 \div 5 = 1$. Back to the whole. Magic!

TIME TO TRY

(a) $\dfrac{2}{3} + \dfrac{1}{3} =$ _____

(b) $\dfrac{5}{8} + \dfrac{3}{8} =$ _____

(c) $\dfrac{7}{11} + \dfrac{4}{11} =$ _____

(d) $\dfrac{3}{4} + \dfrac{1}{4} =$ _____

(e) $\dfrac{5}{10} + \dfrac{4}{10} =$ _____

(f) $\dfrac{6}{12} + \dfrac{5}{12} =$ _____

Answers: (a) 1 (b) 1 (c) 1 (d) 1 (e) 9/10 (f) 11/12.

If you need more practice, there are further examples at the end of the chapter.

APPLYING THE THEORY

Surveys and reports often use fractions to describe the results of the investigation being undertaken. It is really important that you are able to check that what is being claimed matches the data presented, so that you can make well-structured arguments in your assignments. You may find that when you add the fractions together, they do not do add up to one. You need to question the data.

> **KEY POINTS**
> - The numerator is divided by the denominator in vulgar fractions.
> - The denominator shows the number of parts into which the whole has been broken.
> - The numerator tells you how many parts are being used.

So far you have seen examples where the denominators are the same for each fraction. The rule for adding these is just to add the numerators and place them over the denominator.

Equivalent fractions

Think about the following fractions:

$$\frac{2}{4} \qquad \frac{3}{6} \qquad \frac{4}{8} \qquad \frac{5}{10}$$

These all have different denominators, but are **equivalent fractions** – they all have the same value of 1/2. Don't believe it? Look at **Figure 2.3**.

The pies (a)–(d) are equal in size and you can see that each fraction occupies the same amount of space as shown by the tinted area on the right of each diagram.

To prove that they are equivalent, they can be simplified and made more user-friendly by simplifying or 'cancelling'.

The first step is to find a number that divides into both the top and bottom numbers. *Whatever you do to the top line you must do the same to the bottom.*

In all these fractions, the numerator can be divided by itself, making 1 on the top. The denominator can be divided by the numerator with the answer 2. All the fractions are reduced to 1/2. Although these all have different numerators and denominators, they are equivalent fractions – they all have the same value of 1/2.

These are straightforward examples and you could probably see that the denominator is twice the numerator.

Look at the following examples.

$$\text{(a)} \ \frac{7}{21} \qquad \text{(b)} \ \frac{15}{45}$$

Find numbers that divide into both the top and bottom figures and cancel the original number and put in the new one:

(a) $\dfrac{7^1}{21^3}$ Seven divides into both numbers so the fraction is reduced to $\dfrac{1}{3}$.

(b) $\dfrac{15^3}{45^9}$ Five divides into both numbers to give $\dfrac{3}{9}$. This can be further reduced.

Three divides into both numbers $\dfrac{3^1}{9^3}$ to give $\dfrac{1}{3}$.

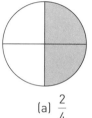 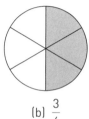 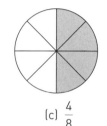 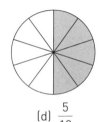

(a) $\dfrac{2}{4}$ (b) $\dfrac{3}{6}$ (c) $\dfrac{4}{8}$ (d) $\dfrac{5}{10}$

Figure 2.3 Equivalent fractions

You might also have noticed that both numbers could be divided by 15 and you would end up with the same answer. Just do the calculation in the way that makes you feel confident. Use as many stages as you need.

TIME TO TRY

Which fraction in each of the following is not equivalent?

1. (a) 1/2   (b) 2/4   (c) 3/7   (d) 5/10

2. (a) 1/3   (b) 3/6   (c) 3/9   (d) 4/12

3. (a) 2/2   (b) 15/15   (c) 10/10   (d) 11/12

4. (a) 24/36   (b) 6/9   (c) 30/60   (d) 8/12

Answers: 1. (c) (the others = 1/2) **2.** (b) (the others = 1/3) **3.** (d) (the others = 1) **4.** (c) (the others = 2/3).

If you need more practice, there are further examples at the end of the chapter.

APPLYING THE THEORY

You are asked to apply a bandage to a patient's leg. The nurse in charge says that you should overlap the layers by 1/2. The next day you are asked by another nurse to apply the bandage and to overlap it by 3/6. Are you confused about which is the correct way to put the bandage on the patient's leg? You shouldn't be, because they are equivalent fractions: 3/6 can be simplified to 1/2.

> ### KEY POINT
> - When simplifying or cancelling fractions, you must divide both the denominator and the numerator by the same number.

Large numbers are just as straightforward. It doesn't matter how you get to your answer as long as it is the correct one and that you understand the underlying principles.

Small steps make the sum more manageable and help you to understand what you are doing. The following example shows that you can use small divisors that are easier to use to get your answer. Find a number that divides into both the top and bottom numbers. Cancel the original number and replace it with the quotient.

Simplify this fraction

$$\frac{1750}{7000}$$

Handy tips

Any number ending in 0 can be divided by 10, 5 or 2. You can choose which to do.

(a) If you divide each number by 2, your answer is

$$\frac{\cancel{1750}^{875}}{\cancel{7000}^{3500}}$$

(b) If you decide to use 5, then the answer is

$$\frac{\cancel{1750}^{350}}{\cancel{7000}^{1400}}$$

(c) Using 10 the answer is

$$\frac{\cancel{1750}^{175}}{\cancel{7000}^{700}}$$

Each of these answers can be further simplified. *Any* number ending in 5 or 0 can be divided by 5. Divide the numerator and denominator in each of the answers above by 5. You should now have the following:

(a) $\dfrac{175}{700}$ (b) $\dfrac{70}{280}$ (c) $\dfrac{35}{140}$

You can see that they can each be divided by 5 again, so do that now. Your answers should be the following:

(a) $\dfrac{35}{140}$ (b) $\dfrac{14}{56}$ (c) $\dfrac{7}{28}$

Looking at these fractions again, you can see that there is still room for further reduction. Fraction (a) can be divided by 5, (b) by 2 or 7 and (c) by 7. If you try this, you will get

(a) $\dfrac{7}{28}$ (b) $\dfrac{7}{28}$ or $\dfrac{1}{4}$ (c) $\dfrac{1}{4}$

You should be able to see now that the answer to all of these will eventually be 1/4 and that it doesn't matter which way you do the calculation, the answer will be the same. It is easier to think about doing a calculation using 1/4 rather than 1750/7000.

More handy tips

Dividing by 3 or 9

If the digits in a number are added together and the sum can be divided by 3, then the number is as well, e.g. 1854.

Add the digits together: $1 + 8 + 5 + 4 = 18$. Then $1 + 8 = 9$ and 9 can be divided by 3, so 1854 can also be divided by 3.

The same method can also be used to see if a number can be divided by 9.

Dividing by 4

If the last two digits of a number are 00 or the number formed by the last two digits is divisible by 4, then the number itself can be divided by 4, e.g. 100 is divisible by 4. The number 3 783 640 512 ends in 12 and it is divisible by 4, so the whole number can be divided by 4. (This is also useful in working out which years are leap years.)

Prime numbers

There are some numbers that can only be divided by 1 and the number itself, with no remainder. This means that sometimes there is no way to make them any simpler. These are called prime numbers (**Table 2.1**).

Table 2.1 Prime numbers up to 101

2	3	5	7	11	13	17	19	23	29	31	37	41
43	47	53	59	61	67	71	73	79	83	89	97	101

TIME TO TRY

Now look at these fractions and use the same method to reduce each to the smallest possible fraction. (Don't forget the handy tips to help choose your divisor.)

(a) $\dfrac{36}{108}$ (b) $\dfrac{125}{375}$ (c) $\dfrac{81}{243}$

These are also equivalent fractions and you should have cancelled them down to 1/3. You have a choice of numbers that will divide into both the numerator and denominator.

If you need more practice, there are further examples at the end of the chapter

APPLYING THE THEORY

Vulgar fractions are sometimes encountered in the calculation of drug doses so it is useful to be able to do them quickly and accurately. Having confidence in your ability to carry out the calculations will free you up to concentrate on other aspects of drug administration.

What if?

So far you have added fractions with the same denominator or have equivalent fractions that can be changed to the same by simplifying. What happens when the numbers of the denominator are not the same?

You change them to equivalent fractions so that the denominators become the same. We say that they have a **common denominator**. Consider

$$\frac{2}{5} + \frac{1}{2}$$

To do this you need to find a number that can be divided by both denominators. In this case, both 5 and 2 can divide into 10, so you can make both fractions into tenths.

To change fifths to tenths, the fraction has to be multiplied by 2.

You have already seen that one of the rules of arithmetic is that whatever change is made to the denominator has to be applied to the numerator.

Following this rule, both 2 and 5 are multiplied by 2 to give 4/10, equivalent to 2/5.

Halves can be changed to tenths by multiplying both parts of the fraction by 5, so 1/2 becomes the equivalent fraction 5/10.

Now both fractions are in tenths, they can be added easily:

$$\frac{4}{10} + \frac{5}{10} = \frac{9}{10}$$

Let's look at a couple more examples of adding fractions with different denominators:

$$\frac{1}{6} + \frac{3}{4}$$

First find the common denominator. What number can be divided by both 6 and 4?

The quickest way to find it is to multiply the denominators of the fractions together, which in this case is $6 \times 4 = 24$. This is not the lowest common denominator but is fine if the numbers involved are small. A better choice would be 12, but it makes no difference to the answer.

Now set out the sum like this:

$$\frac{1}{6} + \frac{3}{4} = \frac{2 + 9}{12} = \frac{11}{12}$$

If you had chosen 24 as your common denominator, then the sum would be

$$\frac{4 + 18}{24} = \frac{22}{24}$$

The answer can be simplified to 11/12 which is the same answer as before.

TIME TO TRY

Remember to find the common denominator first.

(a) 1/3 + 1/4 = _____   (b) 2/7 + 1/2 = _____   (c) 1/5 + 2/3 = _____

(d) 3/8 + 1/2 = _____   (e) 4/7 + 1/3 = _____   (f) 1/10 + 4/5 = _____

Answers: (a) 7/12 (b) 11/14 (c) 13/15 (d) 7/8 (e) 19/21 (f) 9/10.

If you need more practice, there are further examples at the end of the chapter.

So far we have had fractions where the numerator is less than the denominator, but of course this cannot be the case all the time. A fraction that has a numerator of greater value than the denominator is called an **improper fraction**.

When you are adding fractions, and the answer ends up as an improper fraction, the answer has to be simplified:

$$\frac{3}{5} + \frac{4}{5} = \frac{7}{5}$$

You will remember that 7/5 means 7 divided by 5 so you have 1 and 2/5 over.

The answer is written as $1\frac{2}{5}$. This number is called a **mixed number** because it is a combination of whole numbers and fractions. If you had an answer such as 11/5, then it would be simplified to $2\frac{1}{5}$.

You may also have calculations that involve the addition of mixed numbers. For example,

$$3\frac{3}{4} + 2\frac{2}{3}$$

The first thing to do is to change the mixed numbers into improper fractions. Multiply the whole number by the numerator of the fraction and then add the numerator of the fraction to the answer.

In the above sum $3 \times 4 = 12$ (12 quarters) and add the numerator $12 + 3$.

This makes the improper fraction 15/4 (you can check this by changing it back to a mixed number).

The other mixed number is treated in the same way: $2 \times 3 = 6$ and $6 + 2 = 8$, so the other improper fraction is 8/3.

We can now add the two improper fractions together in the usual way by finding the common denominator:

$$\frac{15}{4} + \frac{8}{3}$$

$$\frac{(3 \times 15) + (4 \times 8)}{12}$$

$$= \frac{45 + 32}{12}$$

$$= \frac{77}{12}$$

Simplify this improper fraction to a mixed number by dividing 77 by 12, which gives the answer $6\frac{5}{12}$.

TIME TO TRY

(a) $2\frac{1}{4} + 1\frac{1}{2} =$ _____

(b) $3\frac{1}{8} + 2\frac{1}{4} =$ _____

(c) $1\frac{5}{8} + 4\frac{1}{2} =$ _____

(d) $5\frac{3}{5} + 3\frac{7}{10} =$ _____

(e) $1\frac{1}{3} + 6\frac{1}{6} =$ _____

(f) $7\frac{1}{3} + 2\frac{5}{9} =$ _____

Answers: (a) $3\frac{3}{4}$ (b) $5\frac{3}{8}$ (c) $6\frac{1}{8}$ (d) $9\frac{3}{10}$ (e) $7\frac{1}{2}$ (f) $9\frac{8}{9}$.

If you need more practice, there are further examples at the end of the chapter.

2.2 SUBTRACTION OF VULGAR FRACTIONS

Now that you have mastered addition of fractions, subtraction is easy.

YOUR STARTING POINT FOR SUBTRACTION OF VULGAR FRACTIONS

Without using a calculator, write down the answers to the following in their *simplest form*.

(a) 3/4 − 1/2 = _____ (b) 2/3 − 1/6 = _____ (c) 3/8 − 1/4 = _____

(d) 5/12 − 1/3 = _____ (e) 3/10 − 1/6 = _____ (f) 4/5 − 1/5 = _____

(g) $2\frac{1}{3} - 1\frac{5}{8}$ = _____ (h) $3\frac{3}{4} - 2\frac{2}{3}$ = _____ (i) $6\frac{1}{9} - 5\frac{2}{5}$ = _____

Answers: (a) 1/4 (b) 1/2 (c) 1/8 (d) 1/12 (e) 2/15 (f) 3/5 (g) 17/24 (h) $1\frac{1}{12}$ (i) 32/45.

If you had all these correct answers, go to Section 2.3, the starting point for multiplication and division of fractions.

If you struggled with these or need to be more confident, then work through the parts of the following section that you feel you need.

The principles of finding a common denominator are used again when subtracting fractions. Also remember the rules from Chapter 1 about which number is subtracted from which.

If you look at a simple example, you will see that the layout is familiar:

$$\frac{1}{2} - \frac{1}{4}$$

You may well be able to do this in your head and get the answer 1/4, but it is a good place to start so that you can see the way in which you can tackle calculations when the answer is not immediately obvious. Don't panic when the numbers look too big to handle. Write down this simple sum and then work out the one that may be a problem beside it and follow the steps.

Just as you did with the addition, you first need to find a common denominator, which in this case is 4. Now divide the denominator of each fraction in turn into the common denominator so that you can make equivalent fractions, just as you did when adding fractions. You then subtract the results.

$$\frac{1}{2} - \frac{1}{4}$$
$$= \frac{2 - 1}{4}$$
$$= \frac{1}{4}$$

Subtraction of any vulgar fraction is done in the same way.

TIME TO TRY

Give the answers to the following in the simplest form.

(a) 3/4 − 1/2 = _____   (b) 1/2 − 1/3 = _____

(c) 4/9 − 1/4 = _____   (d) 3/5 − 1/10 = _____

(e) 21/24 − 5/12 = _____   (f) 7/10 − 3/5 = _____

Answers: (a) 1/4 (b) 1/6 (c) 7/36 (d) 1/2 (e) 11/24 (f) 1/10.

If you need more practice, there are further examples at the end of the chapter.

If you have mixed numbers, then you treat them in the same way as you did when you did the addition. First, change the mixed numbers to improper fractions, then find the common denominator and work from there as in this example:

$$3\frac{2}{3} - 2\frac{1}{9}$$

$$= \frac{11}{3} - \frac{19}{9}$$

$$= \frac{33 - 19}{9}$$

Now simplify to a mixed number

$$= \frac{14}{9} = 1\frac{5}{9}$$

TIME TO TRY

(a) $1\frac{2}{3} - 1\frac{1}{4}$ = _____   (b) $3\frac{1}{2} - 2\frac{7}{8}$ = _____   (c) $9\frac{1}{4} - 4\frac{3}{5}$ = _____

(d) $5\frac{9}{10} - 3\frac{1}{2}$ = _____   (e) $4\frac{1}{9} - 3\frac{2}{3}$ = _____   (f) $6\frac{5}{7} - 3\frac{1}{4}$ = _____

Answers: (a) 5/12 (b) 5/8 (c) $4\frac{13}{20}$ (d) $2\frac{2}{5}$ (e) 4/9 (f) $3\frac{13}{28}$.

If you need more practice, there are further examples at the end of the chapter.

As you have now found, subtraction and addition of fractions is straightforward if you remember the key points.

KEY POINTS

When adding or subtracting fractions:

- First, change any mixed numbers to improper fractions.
- Find the common denominator.
- Give the answer in its simplest form.

2.3 MULTIPLICATION AND DIVISION OF VULGAR FRACTIONS

YOUR STARTING POINT FOR MULTIPLICATION AND DIVISION OF VULGAR FRACTIONS

Without using a calculator, write down the answers to the following in their *simplest form*.

(a) 1/2 × 2/5 = _____   (b) 1/7 × 3/4 = _____   (c) 2/3 × 3/5 = _____

(d) 2/5 × 3/4 = _____   (e) 9/10 × 2/5 = _____   (f) $2\frac{1}{3} \times 1\frac{3}{5}$ = _____

(g) 2/3 ÷ 1/2 = _____   (h) 4/5 ÷ 1/4 = _____   (i) 3/5 ÷ 3/4 = _____

(j) 1/2 ÷ 1/4 = _____   (k) 3/4 ÷ 2/7 = _____   (l) $3\frac{1}{3} \div 2\frac{2}{5}$ = _____

Answers: (a) 1/5 (b) 3/28 (c) 6/15 (d) 3/10 (e) 9/25 (f) $3\frac{11}{15}$ (g) $1\frac{1}{3}$ (h) $3\frac{1}{5}$ (i) 4/5 (j) 2 (k) $2\frac{5}{8}$ (l) $1\frac{7}{18}$.

If you feel confident about all these examples, go to Section 2.4 for the addition and subtraction of **decimal fractions**.

Multiplication of vulgar fractions

Multiplication of fractions is straightforward – honestly. You just multiply the numerators together, then multiply the denominators together and simplify the answer, if necessary.

Look at this example:

$$\frac{1}{2} \times \frac{2}{3} = \frac{2}{6}$$

The answer can be simplified to 1/3.

If the calculation involves mixed numbers, then you do as you did in the addition and subtraction sections. Change the numbers to improper fractions, and then multiply.

Work through this example:

$$2\frac{2}{3} \times 1\frac{3}{8}$$

Change these mixed numbers to improper fractions:

$$\frac{8}{3} \times \frac{11}{8}$$

Multiply the numerators together $\dfrac{8 \times 11}{3 \times 8} = \dfrac{88}{24}$
Multiply the denominators together

Simplify the answer by dividing the numerator and denominator by 8:

$$\frac{88^{11}}{24_3} = \frac{11}{3} = 3\frac{2}{3}$$

If you are multiplying a fraction by a whole number on its own, it is safer to put 1 as the denominator so that you do not mistakenly use it as a numerator. (Did you remember that any number divided or multiplied by 1 remains unchanged?) For example,

$$3 \times \frac{4}{5} = \frac{3}{1} \times \frac{4}{5} = \frac{12}{5} = 2\frac{2}{5}$$

TIME TO TRY

(a) $2/5 \times 4/7 =$ _____

(b) $1/3 \times 3/5 =$ _____

(c) $7/10 \times 3/7 =$ _____

(d) $2\frac{1}{2} \times 4\frac{1}{4} =$ _____

(e) $2\frac{2}{3} \times 1\frac{1}{10} =$ _____

(f) $4\frac{2}{5} \times 10/11 =$ _____

Answers: (a) 8/35 (b) 1/5 (c) 3/10 (d) $10\frac{5}{8}$ (e) $2\frac{14}{15}$ (f) 4.

If you need more practice, there are further examples at the end of the chapter.

> **KEY POINTS**
>
> When multiplying vulgar fractions you need to:
> - First change any mixed numbers to improper fractions.
> - Multiply the numerators together.
> - Multiply the denominators.
> - Simplify the answer.

Division of vulgar fractions

You have already come across the idea of division of fractions at the beginning of the chapter. Fractions are already a division of a whole. You saw that one cake was divided into five parts which were called fifths and written as 1/5.

Division of fractions is carried out in a similar way to multiplication except that the second fraction is turned upside down (**inverted**) and then the two fractions are multiplied.

After inverting the second fraction, you can simplify before multiplying. Smaller numbers are easier to use, but, again, use the method that suits you best.

EXAMPLE

$$\frac{2}{3} \div \frac{1}{2}$$

This could also be written as

$$\frac{\frac{2}{3}}{\frac{1}{2}}$$

This is quite clumsy but underlies the reason for inverting the dividing fraction (see website at the end of the chapter).

First, invert the second fraction and replace the division sign with a multiplication one:

$$\frac{2}{3} \times \frac{2}{1}$$

Multiply the numerators and denominators $= \frac{4}{3}$

Now simplify to a mixed number $= 1\frac{1}{3}$

You can apply the method that you used for multiplying mixed numbers to division problems.

EXAMPLE

$$3\frac{1}{3} \div 2\frac{2}{7}$$

Change to improper fractions $\quad = \frac{10}{3} \div \frac{16}{7}$

Invert the second fraction and replace the division sign with a multiplication one

$$= \frac{\cancel{10}^{5}}{3} \times \frac{7}{\cancel{16}^{8}}$$

$$= \frac{35}{24} = 1\frac{11}{24}$$

In this case you can simplify the sum to make multiplication easier. Remember that whatever you do to the denominator is done to the numerator. It doesn't matter which denominator or numerator is simplified.

TIME TO TRY

(a) 3/7 ÷ 1/3 = _____

(b) 1/5 ÷ 1/4 = _____

(c) 11/10 ÷ 1/20 = _____

(d) $2\frac{1}{2} \div 1\frac{1}{4}$ = _____

(e) $3\frac{1}{3} \div 2\frac{2}{3}$ = _____

(f) $3\frac{5}{7} \div 2\frac{1}{6}$ = _____

Answers: (a) $1\frac{2}{7}$ (b) 4/5 (c) 22 (d) 2 (e) $1\frac{1}{4}$ (f) $1\frac{5}{7}$.

If you need more practice, there are further examples at the end of the chapter.

KEY POINTS

When dividing vulgar fractions:

- First change any mixed numbers to improper fractions.
- Invert (turn upside down) the second fraction.
- Multiply the numerators.
- Multiply the denominators.
- Simplify the answer.

2.4 ADDITION AND SUBTRACTION OF DECIMAL FRACTIONS

YOUR STARTING POINT FOR ADDITION AND SUBTRACTION OF DECIMAL FRACTIONS

Add the following decimal fractions.

(a) 0.28 + 0.74 = _____   (b) 2.62 + 0.77 = _____

(c) 1.725 + 2.15 = _____

Subtract the following fractions.

(d) 3.25 − 1.34 = _____   (e) 3.55 − 2.49 = _____

(f) 9.543 − 3.45 = _____

Answers: (a) 1.02 (b) 3.39 (c) 3.875 (d) 1.19 (e) 1.06 (f) 6.093.

If you have answered all these correctly, congratulations. Move on to multiplication and division, Section 2.5.

Decimal fractions

You are already very familiar with decimal fractions since you use them every time you go shopping. A pound and thirty-one pence can be written as £1.31. Pence are a decimal fraction of a pound.

In Chapter 1 we saw the importance of place value and used columns to indicate units, tens, hundreds, thousands and so on.

The decimal point marks the division between whole numbers and decimal fractions. These fractions are tenths, hundredths, thousandths and so on.

It is vital that you are clear about the placement of the decimal point in the number. There is only one decimal place difference between £1.31 and £13.10 but you have 10 times as much money when you have £13.10.

LOOK OUT

You need to make sure that when you give drugs that you are certain of the position of the decimal point, otherwise you can give a patient 10 times the prescribed dose.

Writing and saying decimal fractions

In the number 3214.759, you can see from **Table 2.2** that the figures to the left of the decimal point are the whole numbers and those to the right are the decimal fractions. This number represents 3000 + 200 + 10 + 4 before the decimal point, and 7/10, 5/100 and 9/1000 to the right of the decimal point.

Table 2.2

Thousands	Hundreds	Tens	Units	Decimal point	Tenths	Hundredths	Thousandths
3	2	1	4	•	7	5	9

It is accepted practice when saying the decimal part of the number to say each individual figure rather than saying seven hundred and fifty-nine, so that there is no confusion with whole numbers.

When we write whole numbers the decimal point is not used, but you should remember that it is there in theory to the right of the figure, e.g. we write 5 or 17 rather than 5.0 or 17.0.

APPLYING THE THEORY

Many clinical measurements and calculations involve decimal fractions. Body temperature is measured in degrees Celsius. Normal temperature is 37°C but there is a significant difference between 37°C and 38°C so each degree is divided into tenths so that a temperature can be recorded more accurately, e.g. 37.6°C.

Adding and subtracting decimals

Addition and subtraction of decimals is very little different from addition and subtraction of whole numbers that you did in Chapter 1.

It is important to align the decimal points under each other. Just as you did with whole numbers, you start the sum from the figure furthest to the right.

EXAMPLES

(a) 2.23 + 0.65   2.23
                  +0.65
                  ‾‾‾‾‾
                   2.88

(b) 1.735 + 2.3   1.735
                 +2.300
                 ‾‾‾‾‾‾
                  4.035

You may find it helpful to put zeros in spaces to keep decimal columns aligned as in 2.3 in example (b) above.

Subtraction of decimal fractions is also similar to the subtraction of whole numbers. As with addition, you need to make sure that you keep the decimal points under each other.

EXAMPLES

$$2.39 - 1.27$$

$$\begin{array}{r} 2.39 \\ -1.27 \\ \hline 1.12 \end{array}$$

$$4.35 - 3.72$$

$$\begin{array}{r} {}^{3}4.{}^{1}36 \\ -3.72 \\ \hline 0.64 \end{array}$$

TIME TO TRY

(a) 3.51 + 2.38 = _____

(b) 7.87 + 2.34 = _____

(c) 21.045 + 10.945 = _____

(d) 2.25 − 1.13 = _____

(e) 3.63 − 1.42 = _____

(f) 12.43 − 9.58 = _____

Answers: (a) 5.89 (b) 10.21 (c) 31.99 (d) 1.12 (e) 2.21 (f) 2.85.

If you need more practice, there are further examples at the end of the chapter.

KEY POINT

● When adding and subtracting decimal fractions, they are done in the same way as whole numbers, except that the decimal points must be aligned.

2.5 MULTIPLICATION AND DIVISION OF DECIMAL FRACTIONS

YOUR STARTING POINT FOR MULTIPLICATION AND DIVISION OF DECIMAL FRACTIONS

Change the vulgar fractions to decimal fractions correct to two decimal places.

(a) 2/9 = _____

(b) 3/7 = _____

(c) 4/9 = _____

Multiply the following:

(d) 7.5 × 3.4 = _____

(e) 5.92 × 6.8 = _____

(f) 24.43 × 11.94 = _____

Divide the following:

(g) 4.2 ÷ 1.5 = _____

(h) 3.95 ÷ 1.5 = _____

(i) 14.44 ÷ 1.2 = _____

Answers: (a) 0.22 (b) 0.43 (c) 0.44 (d) 25.50 (e) 40.26 (f) 291.69 (g) 2.80 (h) 2.63 (i) 12.03.

If you are happy with your answers, go to Section 2.6, read the section on exponents and do the calculations.

Multiplication of decimal fractions

You are now going to apply your knowledge of multiplication from Chapter 1.

Do you remember how to multiply whole numbers by 10?

Multiply each of these numbers by 10, 100, 1000. (*Hint:* 100 = 10 × 10 and 1000 = 10 × 10 × 10.)

(a) 2 × 10 = _____ 2 × 100 = _____ 2 × 1000 = _____

(b) 23 × 10 = _____ 23 × 100 = _____ 23 × 1000 = _____

(c) 145 × 10 = _____ 145 × 100 = _____ 145 × 1000 = _____

Answers: (a) 20, 200, 2000 (b) 230, 2300, 23 000 (c) 1450, 14 500, 145 000.

You will have noticed the pattern. To multiply by 10, add one zero, by 100 add two zeros and by 1000 add three zeros. The numbers get bigger as the place value changes.

When multiplying decimal fractions by 10, 100 and 1000, rather than adding zeros you move the decimal point the same number of places to the *right* as there are zeros. Again the number becomes bigger.

Look at the following example:

$$0.142 \times 10 = 1.42 \qquad 0.142 \times 100 = 14.2 \qquad 0.142 \times 1000 = 142$$

Write out the answer to this sum

$$0.142 \times 10\,000 = \underline{\hspace{1cm}}$$

You need to move the decimal point. How many places? Four. But there are not enough numbers so you have to add a zero to ensure place value is maintained.

$$0 \cdot 142 \times 10 \quad 1 \cdot 42 \times 10 \quad 14 \cdot 2 \times 10 \quad 142 \cdot 0 \times 10 \quad 1420$$

So your answer is 1420.

 Chapter 3 – conversion of units.

TIME TO TRY

(a) 2.7 × 10 = _____   (b) 45.1 × 1000 = _____

(c) 345.25 × 100 = _____   (d) 12.3 × 10 000 = _____

(e) 5.1 × 1 000 000 = _____   (f) 19.4 × 100 = _____

Answers: (a) 27 (b) 45 100 (c) 34 525 (d) 123 000 (e) 5 100 000 (f) 1940.

If you need more practice, there are further examples at the end of the chapter.

APPLYING THE THEORY

It is vital that you are confident in multiplying by 10, 100 and 1000. Many drug calculations, physiological measurements and fluid measurements involve multiplying and dividing by these numbers.

You do not need to worry about the decimal point when you are multiplying two decimal fractions together. The important thing is that you put the decimal point in the correct place at the end of the calculation.

It doesn't matter which number is multiplied by which (I usually multiply by the smaller one as it often has fewer figures to multiply).

EXAMPLE

$$23.4 \times 3.8$$

Take out the decimal points and treat it like a normal multiplication. (What you are really doing is multiplying each number by 10 so that the decimal point is moved so far that you are left with a whole number.)

$$
\begin{array}{r}
234 \\
\times \quad 38 \\
\hline
7020 \\
1872 \\
\hline
8892 \\
\end{array}
$$

Now you can consider the position of the decimal point.

The rule is that the answer to the sum must have the same number of decimal places as the *total* in the numbers multiplied together. In this case, both 23.4 and 3.8 have one decimal place, so the answer must have two decimal places. (What you are doing now is reversing the multiplication by 10 and 10 that you used to get rid of the decimal points. You are now dividing by 10 and 10 or 100.)

So $23.4 \times 3.8 = 88.92$. It is useful to have a rough idea of the answer as this will help with checking the place of the decimal point. In this case $23 \times 4 = 92.0$ which is close to your answer of 88.92.

Use the above information to follow the working of this example:

$$
\begin{array}{r}
4.7 \times 3.25 = 325 \\
\times \ 47 \\
\hline
13\,000 \\
2\,275 \\
\hline
15\,275 \\
\end{array}
$$

The original sum had a total of three decimal places, so the answer needs three decimal places. You multiplied the first number by 10 and the second number by 100, so you need to move the decimal point three places from the right.

The answer is 15.275. Is this a sensible answer?

TIME TO TRY

(a) 4.2 × 3.6 = _____

(b) 3.5 × 1.2 = _____

(c) 6.4 × 4.25 = _____

(d) 2.56 × 5.9 = _____

(e) 21.35 × 1.25 = _____

(f) 2.72 × 2.43 = _____

Answers: (a) 15.12 (b) 4.2 (c) 27.2 (d) 15.104 (e) 26.6875 (f) 6.6096.

If you need more practice, there are further examples at the end of the chapter.

Division of decimal fractions

Division of decimals is just like division of whole numbers except that we don't have a remainder if the numbers don't divide exactly. The number of decimal places, in theory, is unlimited but the number of places is restricted in everyday life to manageable limits.

We will start off with division of whole numbers by 10, 100 and 1000. You are already familiar with multiplication by these numbers and division is just as straightforward. When you divide a number, you expect your answer to be smaller:

$$5000 \div 10 = 500 \quad 5000 : 100 = 50 \quad 5000 \div 1000 = 5$$

Again a pattern is emerging. It seems that the number of zeros removed from 5000 is the same number of zeros in the divisor – one when dividing by 10, two when dividing by 100 and three with 1000.

Think about what is happening. We said earlier that in whole numbers the decimal point is not usually shown but in theory is after the last figure. You can then see that when 5000 is divided by 10, the decimal point moves one place to the left, making the number smaller. When divided by 100 the decimal point moves two places to the left and three places when divided by 1000.

Now try this one:

$$5000 \div 10\,000 = \underline{\hspace{2cm}}$$

How many places do you need to move the decimal point? It might help if you put the decimal point in. That is,

$$5000 \cdot 0 \div 10 \quad 500 \cdot 0 \div 10 \quad 50 \cdot 0 \div 10 \quad 5 \cdot 0 \div 10 \quad 0 \cdot 5$$

So your answer is 0.5.

 Chapter 3 – conversion of units.

TIME TO TRY

(a) 2.7 ÷ 10 = _____

(b) 45.1 ÷ 1000 = _____

(c) 345.25 ÷ 100 = _____

(d) 1234 ÷ 10000 = _____

(e) 5 000 000 ÷ 1 000 000 = _____

(f) 1945 ÷ 100 = _____

If you need more practice, there are further examples at the end of the chapter.

Vulgar fractions can be easily changed to the decimal equivalent by dividing the numerator into the denominator.

A half is written as 1/2 as a vulgar fraction and 0.5 as a decimal fraction; 1/2 means 1 divided by 2 (1 ÷ 2).

This is a straightforward example, in which you may not have even considered how one is changed to the other.

You treat it like a long-division sum. Go back to Chapter 1 if you need to refresh your memory (page 22). Now 2 divided into 1 won't go, so you put a zero and a decimal point on the line and a decimal point after the 1 and add a zero. You now have 2 dividing into 10, which goes five times, so you put 5 on the line, giving you the answer 0.5:

$$2\overline{)1.^10} \quad \begin{array}{c} 0.5 \end{array}$$

Another straightforward example:

1/4 means 1 divided by 4 $\quad 4\overline{)1.0^20} \quad \begin{array}{c} 0.25 \end{array}$

You need to take care that the decimal point of the quotient is above the decimal point of the dividend, otherwise you might make a mistake in your calculation.

When you are dividing numbers to make them into decimal fractions, you may find that you could keep on dividing and have 10 or more numbers after the decimal point. This is not usually practical so we need to know how accurate the calculation needs to be. Usually, you need an answer **correct to two decimal places**.

This means that you need to divide until you have three numbers after the decimal point.

You then need to look at the third figure after the decimal point. If it is less than five, then the second number remains the same. If the third figure is five or more, then the second number is increased by 1.

EXAMPLES

(a) 1/3 = 1 ÷ 3 $\quad 3\overline{)1.0^10^10} \quad \begin{array}{c} 0.3\ 3\ 3 \end{array}$

The third figure is less than five, so the answer, correct to two decimal places, is 0.33.

(b) 2/3 = 2 ÷ 3

$$3\overline{)2.0^20^20}$$ 0.6 6 6

The third figure is more than five, so the answer, correct to two decimal places, is 0.67.

> **LOOK OUT**
>
> You will have noticed that there is a zero before the decimal point. It ensures that the figures are a decimal fraction and not whole numbers. A decimal point on its own could easily be missed, which could result in a potentially serious drug error. For example, a patient might receive 100 times the dose if someone mistook 0.25 for 25.

APPLYING THE THEORY

When calculating drug doses, particularly those involving small parts of a normal size dose, you need to ensure how accurate the final dose has to be. It is most common to have the dose correct to one or two decimal places.

In some measurements, such as calculation of fluid intake, there may be no need to be as accurate, so the answer may be correct to the nearest whole number.

You can change any vulgar fraction to a decimal fraction. It is useful to learn the common ones.

Change these vulgar fractions to decimal fractions.

(a) 1/5 = _____   (b) 1/8 = _____   (c) 3/4 = _____

(d) 1/10 = _____   (e) 2/5 = _____   (f) 1/2 = _____

Answers: (a) 0.2 (b) 0.125 (c) 0.75 (d) 0.1 (e) 0.4 (f) 0.5.

You are more than halfway to dividing decimal fractions!

If you need to divide a decimal fraction by another decimal fraction, you first need to put them in a form that is easily manageable.

Look at this example:

$$3.2 ÷ 2.5$$

The first thing to do is to get rid of the decimal point in the divisor so that you have a whole number to carry out the calculation.

To do this you need to multiply both numbers by 10. So

$$3.2 × 10 = 32 \quad \text{and} \quad 2.5 × 10 = 25$$

The sum is now 32 ÷ 25, so you can set it out like an ordinary division, making sure that the decimal points of the dividend and the quotient are kept aligned.

You can set out the sum as you did in Chapter 1:

$$25\overline{)32.^70\ ^{20}0}\qquad 1.2\ \ 8$$

Or like this

```
        1.28
25)32.00
      −25       25 divides into 32 once, remainder 7
       70
      −50       25 into 70 goes twice, remainder 20
      200
     −200       25 into 200 goes eight times exactly
      000
```

Use whichever method you prefer. You do not have to worry about the position of the decimal point because you multiplied both numbers by the same amount, so it will make no difference to the final answer.

Not sure? Think about this example:

$$40 \div 20 = 2$$

Now divide 40 and 20 by 10 to get 4 and 2:

$$4 \div 2 = 2 \quad \text{same answer}$$

TIME TO TRY

Calculate the following, correct to two decimal places.

(a) $2.5 \div 0.5 =$ _____

(b) $3.66 \div 2.4 =$ _____

(c) $43.52 \div 3.2 =$ _____

(d) $42.94 \div 3.8 =$ _____

(e) $5.25 \div 0.75 =$ _____

(f) $26.6 \div 4.2 =$ _____

Answers: (a) 5.00 (b) 1.53 (c) 13.60 (d) 11.30 (e) 7 (f) 6.33.

There are more examples if you need them at the end of the chapter.

APPLYING THE THEORY

Being able to calculate accurately is very important for patient safety. You may have to decide whether you use vulgar or decimal fractions for your calculations. Sometimes it is easier to start off with vulgar fractions and convert the answer to a decimal fraction. The main advantage of working with decimal fractions is that they can be easily checked with a calculator.

> **KEY POINTS**
> - Any vulgar fraction can be converted to a decimal fraction by dividing the numerator by the denominator.
> - When dividing by 10, 100 and 1000, the decimal point is moved to the *left*, making the number *smaller*.
> - If you divide decimal fractions, get rid of the decimal point in the divisor by multiplying it by 10, 100 or a larger multiple of 10. You must remember also to multiply the dividend by the same number.
> - Keep decimal points aligned.

2.6 MORE ABOUT EXPONENTS

In Chapter 1 you learned how exponents can be used to simplify large numbers. Powers of 10 are often used in calculations of physiological measurements. This is called **scientific notation**. You will learn about this in the chapter on physiological measurements.

Do you remember what 10^6 means? It means $10 \times 10 \times 10 \times 10 \times 10 \times 10 = 1\,000\,000$. And

$$\frac{1}{10} \times \frac{1}{10} \times \frac{1}{10} \times \frac{1}{10} \quad \text{can be simplified to} \quad \frac{1}{10^4}.$$

Now $1/10^4$ can also be written as 1×10^{-4} which is said as 'One times 10 to the minus four'. This is called a negative exponent and is another way of saying 1 divided by 10 000.

What would this be as a decimal fraction? _____

Answer: 0.0001.

TIME TO TRY

Write these exponents in full.

(a) $10^3 =$ _____　　　　　(b) $10^8 =$ _____

(c) $10^7 =$ _____　　　　　(d) $10^9 =$ _____

(e) $10^{-3} =$ _____　　　　　(f) $10^{-8} =$ _____

(g) $10^{-7} =$ _____　　　　　(h) $10^{-9} =$ _____

Answers: (a) 1000 (b) 100 000 000 (c) 10 000 000 (d) 1 000 000 000 (e) 0.001 (f) 0.000 000 01 (g) 0.000 000 1 (h) 0.000 000 001.

You will use exponents again with SI units in the next chapter.

You have covered a lot of ground so now is the time to see what you have understood.

> **RUNNING WORDS**
>
> | | | |
> |---|---|---|
> | common denominator | denominator | mixed number |
> | correct to two decimal places | equivalent fractions | numerator |
> | | improper fraction | scientific notation |
> | decimal fractions | inverted | vulgar fractions |

Answers to the following questions can be found at the end of the book.

What did you learn?

(a) Add the following fractions, giving the answer in its simplest form.

(i) 1/3 + 1/3 = _____ (ii) 1/2 + 1/4 = _____

(iii) 1/4 + 1/8 = _____ (iv) 2/3 + 1/6 = _____

(v) 1/5 + 3/10 = _____ (vi) 1/7 + 4/21 = _____

(b) If I divide a cake into 12 equal slices and eat 3 slices, what fraction of the cake is left? Write the answer as a vulgar fraction in its simplest form. _____

(c) A patient uses a glass that holds 1/5 of a jug's volume. The patient drinks eight full glasses during the course of the day. What fraction of the second jug is left at the end of the day? _____

(d) You make a survey of the number of times the staff in the department wash their hands. You find that 1/4 wash their hands three times during the shift, 1/3 four times and the remainder five times. If there is a total of 12 staff, how many people washed their hands five times? _____

(e) A patient's temperature is 39.1°C. You are asked to monitor it regularly after the patient has some medicine to reduce it. You are asked report to the nurse in charge when it has been reduced by 1.5°C because the patient's condition needs to be reviewed. What temperature will be recorded when that point is reached? _____

(f) You work 11.25 hours per week as a care assistant. The hourly rate is £5.45. How much do you earn per week, to the nearest penny? _____

More 'Time to Try' examples

Addition of fractions, page 33

(a) 3/7 + 3/7 = _____   (b) 1/5 + 3/5 = _____

(c) 6/15 + 5/15 = _____   (d) 2/4 + 1/4 = _____

(e) 5/17 + 12/17 = _____   (f) 3/11 + 5/11 = _____

Equivalent fractions, page 35

Which fraction in each of the following is not equivalent?

1. (a) 2/3   (b) 1/7   (c) 4/28   (d) 2/14

2. (a) 1/3   (b) 3/6   (c) 2/4   (d) 9/18

3. (a) 2/3   (b) 10/15   (c) 11/12   (d) 4/6

4. (a) 9/36   (b) 1/6   (c) 3/12   (d) 1/4

Equivalent fractions, page 37
Reduce each of these to the smallest possible fraction.

(a) 45/135 = _____   (b) 80/420 = _____   (c) 42/192 = _____

(d) 144/156 = _____   (e) 14/126 = _____   (f) 39/117 = _____

Equivalent fractions, page 38

(a) 1/4 + 1/3 = _____   (b) 1/2 + 2/7 = _____

(c) 1/6 + 2/3 = _____   (d) 1/8 + 1/2 = _____

(e) 2/7 + 1/3 = _____   (f) 1/10 + 1/5 = _____

Mixed numbers, page 39

(a) $1\frac{1}{4} + 3\frac{1}{2} =$ _____   (b) $2\frac{5}{8} + 1\frac{1}{4} =$ _____

(c) $3\frac{5}{9} + 3\frac{2}{3} =$ _____   (d) $5\frac{3}{10} + 2\frac{1}{5} =$ _____

(e) $6\frac{5}{12} + 1\frac{1}{3} =$ _____   (f) $4\frac{7}{9} + 2\frac{2}{3} =$ _____

Subtraction of fractions, page 41
Give the answers to the following in the simplest form.

(a) 1/4 − 1/5 = _____   (b) 2/3 − 1/2 = _____

(c) 5/9 − 1/6 = _____   (d) 3/10 − 1/5 = _____

(e) 7/12 − 1/36 = _____   (f) 9/20 − 2/5 = _____

Mixed numbers, page 41

(a) $2\frac{1}{3} - 1\frac{1}{4} =$ _____

(b) $2\frac{2}{3} - 1\frac{5}{6} =$ _____

(c) $5\frac{1}{4} - 2\frac{3}{5} =$ _____

(d) $7\frac{3}{10} - 5\frac{1}{2} =$ _____

(e) $4\frac{1}{9} - 3\frac{2}{3} =$ _____

(f) $3\frac{2}{5} - 2\frac{1}{3} =$ _____

Multiplication of fractions, page 43

(a) $3/5 \times 1/4 =$ _____

(b) $1/3 \times 3/4 =$ _____

(c) $3/10 \times 2/3 =$ _____

(d) $3\frac{1}{3} \times 2\frac{1}{4} =$ _____

(e) $2\frac{1}{7} \times 1\frac{1}{3} =$ _____

(f) $2\frac{2}{5} \times 3/10 =$ _____

Division of fractions, page 44

(a) $5/7 \div 1/5 =$ _____

(b) $1/4 \div 1/2 =$ _____

(c) $11/10 \div 1/5 =$ _____

(d) $3\frac{1}{2} \div 1\frac{1}{3} =$ _____

(e) $3\frac{2}{5} \div 1\frac{2}{3} =$ _____

(f) $2\frac{1}{7} \div 3\frac{1}{3} =$ _____

Addition and subtraction of decimal fractions, page 47

(a) $1.72 + 2.14 =$ _____

(b) $8.15 + 2.86 =$ _____

(c) $15.387 + 10.035 =$ _____

(d) $2.28 - 1.15 =$ _____

(e) $4.54 - 1.66 =$ _____

(f) $11.27 - 7.38 =$ _____

Multiplication of decimal fractions, page 48

(a) $3.5 \times 10 =$ _____

(b) $5.7 \times 1000 =$ _____

(c) $3.142 \times 100 =$ _____

(d) $1.49 \times 10\,000 =$ _____

(e) $34.5 \times 1\,000\,000 =$ _____

(f) $1.753 \times 100 =$ _____

Multiplication of decimal fractions, page 50

(a) $2.4 \times 1.7 =$ _____

(b) $4.8 \times 5.4 =$ _____

(c) $1.79 \times 3.45 =$ _____

(d) $6.34 \times 2.8 =$ _____

(e) $3.62 \times 4.19 =$ _____

(f) $2.72 \times 3.1 =$ _____

Division of decimal fractions, page 51

(a) $42.3 \div 10 =$ _____

(b) $3676.1 \div 1000 =$ _____

(c) $3.46 \div 100 =$ _____

(d) $16\,522 \div 10\,000 =$ _____

(e) $4\,302\,225 \div 1\,000\,000 =$ _____

(f) $2008 \div 100 =$ _____

Division of decimal fractions, page 53

Calculate the following, correct to two decimal places.

(a) 2.5 ÷ 1.25 = _____   (b) 4.86 ÷ 2.4 = _____

(c) 81.92 ÷ 3.2 = _____   (d) 461.16 ÷ 36.6 = _____

(e) 0.75 ÷ 1.5 = _____   (f) 93.704 ÷ 3.4_____

Web resources

http://www.helpwithfractions.com
This site covers all aspects of playing with vulgar fractions. In the division section there is an explanation of the reason for inverting the divisor when fractions are divided – if you feel strong. If you can't cope, just accept it!

http://www.mathsisfun.com/fractions_multiplication.html
A step-by-step animated website with plenty of examples for you to do.

http://primes.utm.edu/lists/small/1000.txt
A list of prime numbers that might be useful in finding factors.

http://www.cgpbooks.co.uk/online_rev/ks3/ks3_maths_01.htm
Try the fractions game. Useful for consolidating fractions.

http://www.bbc.co.uk/schools/gcsebitesize/maths/number/
Choose the sections on fractions, although this site is useful for all aspects of maths.

Chapter 3

SI units

How's your French? You only need one phrase: 'Système International d'Unités'

You will need to record patients' temperature, height and weight, measure fluids and give medicines. These are all recorded in special units that have been agreed internationally. You need to be able to carry out calculations using these units.

When you have completed this chapter, you should be able to:

- Identify the units of mass, length, volume.
- Use the units of mass, length and volume and the derived units used in healthcare.
- Demonstrate an understanding of the prefixes used to indicate divisions and multiples of the units.
- Carry out calculations changing units from one to another.
- Identify the hazards in using abbreviations.

It is important that there is a common language when describing mass, length and volume in physiology and healthcare. The Système International d'Unités or SI units was adopted by the UK healthcare system in the early 1970s and is based on the metric system. Some of the metric units had been in common use and established for such a long time that they were kept alongside the new units: for example, the litre and degrees Celsius are used in clinical practice rather than cubic metres and the Kelvin scale for temperature.

Most physiological measurements, patients' vital signs and drug doses rely heavily on a good understanding of SI units and the ability to carry out calculations using these units. The system is used almost everywhere except in the United States, but it is gradually being adopted there.

YOUR STARTING POINT FOR SI UNITS

1. (a) What is the SI unit and its abbreviation used to measure length (distance)? _____

   (b) What is the SI unit and its abbreviation used to measure mass (weight)? _____

   (c) What is the SI unit and its abbreviation used to measure volume? _____

2. Change the following from litres to millilitres or millilitres to litres.

   (a) 1.5 litres = _____ mL   (b) 2 litres = _____ mL

   (c) 250 mL = _____ L   (d) 1245 mL = _____ L

3. Change the following to grams.

   (a) 2 mg = _____   (b) 1000 mg = _____

   (c) 2.4 kg = _____   (d) 1000 micrograms = _____

4. Change the following to kilograms.

   (a) 550 g = _____   (b) 1250 g = _____

   (c) 1250 mg = _____   (d) 35 g = _____

5. Change the following to metres.

   (a) 200 cm = _____   (b) 1 km = _____

   (c) 500 mm = _____   (d) 57 cm = _____

6. Put these values into standard form.

   (a) 2 700 000 = _____   (b) 0.000 013 = _____

   (c) 357.55 = _____   (d) 0.000 783 = _____

7. Change the following to moles or millimoles.

(a) 1.2 mol = _____ mmol   (b) 200 mmol = _____ mol

(c) 0.25 mol = _____ mmol

If you are happy with your results, move on to the questions at the end of the chapter or go through the sections you need to refresh.

3.1 THE UNITS

The standard units cover all types of physical measurement, but the ones that are important in clinical practice are set out in **Table 3.1**.

A weighty problem

The kilogram is the unit used as the measurement of mass. Mass is more common-ly called weight but in scientific terms the two are not exactly the same. Mass is constant but weight varies depending on the effect of gravity, as astronauts discov-er when they go into space.

Kilograms are useful for weighing patients and potatoes but too big for weighing the amount of drug in a tablet. The base unit for medicines is the gram (g) which is 1/1000 of a kilogram. One of the advantages of the divisions of the base units is that they are all a thousand times bigger or smaller than the previous unit (except those shaded ones in Table 3.2 on page 65).

Measuring mass

Mass can be measured with digital scales but often you will use a mechanical triple-**beam balance** (Figure 3.1(a)). The ones that you use in the laboratory measure mass in grams.

Table 3.1 SI base units

Physical quantity	SI unit	Symbol of SI unit
Length	Metre	m
Mass	Kilogram	kg
Volume	Cubic metre	m^3
Amount of substance	Mole	mol
Temperature	Kelvin	K

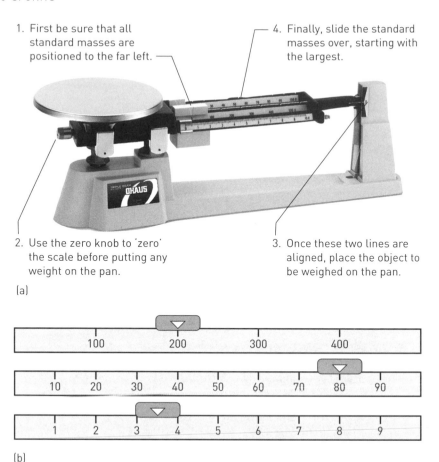

1. First be sure that all standard masses are positioned to the far left.

4. Finally, slide the standard masses over, starting with the largest.

2. Use the zero knob to 'zero' the scale before putting any weight on the pan.

3. Once these two lines are aligned, place the object to be weighed on the pan.

(a)

(b)

Figure 3.1 An example of a triple-beam balance

Source: (a) Ohaus Corporation; (b) Garrett, L., Clarke, A. and Shihab, P. (2008) *Get Ready for A&P for Nursing and Health care*, Pearson Education

Before you use the equipment make sure that all the sliding masses (weights) are pushed as far as possible to the left side of the beams and check that the two lines on the right side are aligned. If they are not, you need to adjust the zero knob until you get alignment when the beam is at rest. *Now* you are ready to measure the mass of your object.

The three beams have a different standard mass. The top one has 100 g divisions, the second 10 g divisions and the third 1 g divisions.

Starting with the 100 g, move the mass along the beam until the arm tips down to the right, then move it back a notch. Move the 10 g mass across until the beam tips and move it back a notch. Finally do the same with the 1 g mass. Read the point at which the arrow meets the scale for each mass, starting with the 100 g beam.

Look at **Figure 3.1(b)**. What is the reading on the scale? _____

Answer: 283.5 g.

APPLYING THE THEORY

Baby weighing scales use the same principles but the scale is in kilograms and grams and the weighing pan is curved to keep the baby safe. Patience is needed to get an accurate reading – wriggling disturbs the balance.

Some adult scales are of similar construction, with a platform to stand on or a seat for those unsteady on their feet.

KEY POINT

● Make sure that the scales are at zero before calculating the mass.

How much space?

Everything takes up space. The amount of space is called the volume. The SI term for volume, **cubic metres**, may not be very familiar. You are probably used to liquids or gases being measured in litres. It is certainly a more manageable unit for every-day practice, since a cubic metre contains a thousand litres!

When liquids are poured into a container, the molecules of the fluid cling to each other and to the wall of the vessel. This is called surface tension and is more obvious in a narrow tube or cylinder. **Surface tension** causes the liquid to climb up the sides of the container, producing a curved surface, lowest in the middle. This is called the **meniscus**. When taking a reading, the bottom of the curve is the reference point that should be used for an accurate measurement (**Figure 3.2**).

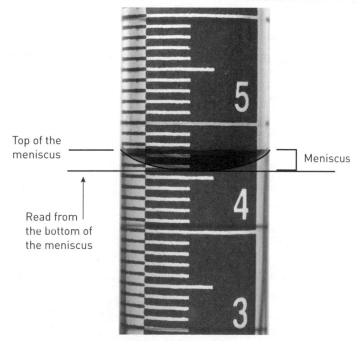

Figure 3.2 Meniscus
© Richard Megna, Fundamental Photographs, NYC

APPLYING THE THEORY

You will have plenty of opportunities to measure volumes in clinical placements. Liquid medicines and injections are obvious examples but you will also need to measure a patient's fluid intake and urinary output in millilitres and litres. Oxygen flow is measured in litres per minute.

> ### LOOK OUT
>
> Liquid medicines are measured in a graduated medicine container. The medicine clings to the side and produces a meniscus, so you must make sure that you read the lower line at eye level to ensure accuracy. These containers are not very precise but the same precautions need to be taken to give the most accurate measure possible.

Surface tension also affects liquids poured into spoons. You can get a heaped spoonful if you pour the liquid slowly. A 5 mL dose in a measuring spoon is level with the rim. There will be more about measuring solutions of drugs in the chapters on the calculating of doses.

How long is a piece of string?

Actually, string is not that useful for measuring as it doesn't have a scale.

The base unit for length is the metre. It is quite a large unit for many of the measurements that you undertake in practice. The height of adults is measured in metres, but for babies and children, centimetres are used. A centimetre is 1/100 of a metre, so there are 100 cm in 1 m.

Look at the centimetre scale of the ruler in **Figure 3.3(a)**. How many millimetres are there in 1 centimetre? (a) _____

Millimetres are used where the data has to be precise, such as measuring the diameters of skin moles. In **Figure 3.3(b)** what is the diameter of the circle? (b) _____

Answers: (a) 10 (b) 44 mm (4.4 cm).

Micrometres and nanometres are used to measure very small anatomical structures such as blood vessels and cells.

The base units are often too large and sometimes too small for accurate measurement, so **prefixes** are used to make fractions or multiples of the standard unit. The ones most commonly used in clinical practice are set out in **Table 3.2**. (The full range of prefixes can be found in Appendix B.)

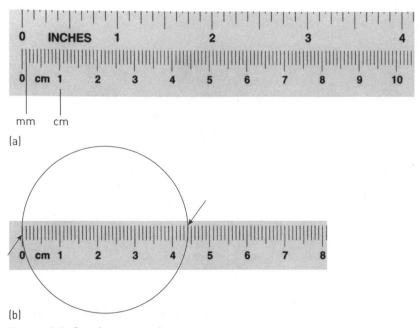

(a)

(b)
Figure 3.3 Centimetre scale
Source: Garrett, L. (2007) *Get Ready for A&P*, Pearson Benjamin Cummings

Table 3.2 Prefixes used in SI units

Prefix	Abbreviation	Multiple or decimal fraction		Exponent	
Giga	G	1 000 000 000		10^9	
Mega	M	1 000 000		10^6	
Kilo	k	1000	Increasing ↑	10^3	
Hecto	h	100		10^2	
Deca	da	10		10^1	
		1	base unit		Vulgar fraction
Deci	d	0.1		10^{-1}	1/10
Centi	c	0.01		10^{-2}	1/100
Milli	m	0.001	Decreasing ↓	10^{-3}	1/1000
Micro	μ	0.000 001		10^{-6}	1/1 000 000
Nano	n	0.000 000 001		10^{-9}	1/1 000 000 000
Pico	p	0.000 000 000 001		10^{-12}	1/1 000 000 000 000
Femto	f	0.000 000 000 000 001		10^{-15}	1/1 000 000 000 000 000

Units in shaded areas are not commonly used in clinical practice, but are included to show how the factors increase or decrease in value.

Abbreviations do not have a plural form (no 's').

 Revisit the sections in Chapters 1 and 2 if you have forgotten how scientific notation and exponents work.

Best guess is not good enough

Many of the opportunities for using these units and their prefixes arise as a result of reading prescriptions and recording drug administration. It is vital that the information is unambiguous in order to avoid drug errors. The abbreviations may be quite clear when printed, but when handwritten can cause confusion.

'Micro' and 'nano' should not be abbreviated. You can imagine that μ and n can look very similar to each other and to the symbol m for 'milli', when handwritten, so to avoid problems they must be written in full.

The abbreviation for litre is officially a lower case L, but since there is a danger of confusion in some print fonts with upper case i (I) or the number 1, it is more usual to use L in print. This form is used throughout the *British National Formulary* which is a reference text that will become very familiar as you progress through your career. It is updated twice a year and you can access the current version of the document via the website reference at the end of the chapter.

LOOK OUT

Avoid confusion. Be clear what units are being used in any measurements in clinical practice. If it is not clear to you, *don't carry on* until you have a satisfactory answer.

KEY POINTS

When writing units in practice:

- Avoid decimal points by converting to a unit giving you whole numbers.
- Micrograms and nanograms should be written in full.
- L is used for litre in print to avoid confusion with the number 1 and capital i (I).

3.2 CHANGING UNITS FROM ONE TO ANOTHER

It is common in clinical practice that the units need to be converted from one size to another, often to avoid decimal points as they can cause confusion. Mistaking the position of the decimal point can result in a patient receiving 10 or 100 times more or less than the prescribed dose.

In Chapter 2 there were some exercises on multiplying and dividing decimal fractions by 10, 100 and 1000. You can now transfer those skills to converting the base units.

- Changing **small** units to **larger** units, you **divide**.
- Changing **large** units to **smaller** units, you **multiply**.

Think about how you change pence to pounds and pounds to pence. The value of £1.00 stays the same if you change it to 100 pence even though you have more individual coins and fewer if you change the small units to the larger one.

Equivalences of weight

1 kilogram (kg) = 1000 grams (g)

1 gram (g) = 1000 milligrams (mg)

1 milligram (mg) = 1000 micrograms (μg); on prescriptions in full – microgram

1 microgram (μg) = 1000 nanograms (ng); on prescriptions in full – nanogram

Equivalences of volume

1 litre (L) = 1000 millilitres (mL)

1 millilitre (mL) = 1000 microlitres (μL); this should be written in full
to prevent confusion with mL

APPLYING THE THEORY

Drug doses are usually relatively small and are commonly prescribed in doses of grams or milligrams. A few drugs need to be given in extremely small doses which are prescribed in micrograms or nanograms.

Liquid medicines are given in small volumes such as 5 mL which is roughly equivalent to a teaspoonful. Children's doses can be even smaller.

Equivalences of length

1 metre (m) = 1000 millimetres (mm)

1 millimetre (mm) = 1000 micrometres

1 micrometre = 1000 nanometres

Centimetres (cm) are often used as a convenient fraction of a metre:

1 metre = 100 centimetres (cm)

1 centimetre = 10 mm

APPLYING THE THEORY

Any type of measurement is useless unless it is done accurately. Whenever you use a measuring device, whether it be a simple tape measure or a complex piece of equipment, you must make sure that it is in working order, it is safe to use, it is accurate and that you understand how it works.

Always ensure that you start your measurement with zero and not one.

You may be asked to measure the length and girth of a patient's leg to ensure that the correct size stockings are ordered. What are the most appropriate units? _____

A baby's length is measured from head to heels in centimetres and along with the baby's weight may be used as part of the calculation for prescribing the correct size drug dose.

Answer: centimetres

67

Some drugs are delivered automatically via a battery-driven syringe. The length of the column of fluid in the syringe is measured in millimetres and the rate adjusted so that the syringe moves at a given number of millimetres per hour. Alignment of the syringe is crucial to accurate measurement. You will learn about these devices in later chapters.

> **KEY POINTS**
>
> - Measurements must be accurate.
> - Understand the equipment you are using.
> - Use appropriate units for the task.

Examples of conversions

Note that zeros are only put in here to make clear how the decimal point is moved.

(a) Change 0.25 g to milligrams

There are 1000 mg in 1 g so you need to *multiply* 0.25 g by 1000. This means that the decimal point has to be moved three places to the *right* (large to small units):

$$0.25 \times 1000 \text{ m} \quad 2 \cdot 50 \quad 25 \cdot 0 \quad 250 \cdot 0 = 250 \text{ mg}$$
$$\times 10 \quad \times 100 \quad \times 1000$$

(b) Change 3.2 mg to micrograms

There are 1000 micrograms in 1 mg.

Again the decimal point is moved three places to the *right* to change a *large to a smaller unit*:

$$3.2 \text{ mg} \times 1000 \quad 32 \cdot 0 \quad 320 \cdot 0 \quad 3200 \cdot 0 = 3200 \text{ micrograms}$$

(c) Change 2750 g to kilograms

There are 1000 g in 1 kg.

This time you are changing a *small unit to a larger one*, so the decimal point is moved three places to the *left*:

$$2750 \text{ g} \div 1000 \quad 275 \cdot 0 \quad 27 \cdot 5 \quad 2 \cdot 75 = 2.75 \text{ kg}$$
$$\div 10 \quad \div 100 \quad \div 1000$$

(d) Change 0.5 L to millilitres

There are 1000 mL in 1 L.

A large unit is being changed to a smaller one, so you have to *multiply* so that the decimal point moves three places to the *right*:

$$0.5 \text{ L} \times 1000 \quad 5 \cdot 0 \quad 50 \cdot 0 \quad 500 \cdot 0 = 500 \text{ mL}$$

(e) Change 0.65 m to centimetres

There are 100 cm in 1 metre.

As with the example above, a large unit is being changed to a smaller one. This time the decimal point is only moved *two* places to the *right* because you only need to multiply by 100:

$$0.65\,\text{m} \times 100 \quad 6{\cdot}5 \quad 65{\cdot}0 = 65\,\text{cm}$$
$$\times 10 \quad \times 100$$

Larger changes

If you need to change units from large units to very small ones, or small to very large, e.g. kilograms to milligrams or nanograms to grams, it is easier to change to the next unit first and then to the next until the size of the unit is reached.

EXAMPLES

(a) Change 2.3 kg to milligrams

First change 2.3 kg to grams:

$$2.3\,\text{kg} \times 1000 = 2300\,\text{g}$$

Now change 2300 g to milligrams:

$$2300\,\text{g} \times 1000 = 2\,300\,000\,\text{mg}$$

There is a convention for presenting numbers in combination with powers of 10, called **standard form**. There is only one number, which must be greater than 0 and less than 10, in front of the decimal point.

If you take 2 300 000 as an example, first put the decimal point immediately after the first number, 2.300 000, and count how many places you have moved the decimal point. In this case it is six to the left. Each place represents dividing by the power of 10.

The zeros do not have any value now, so can be removed. You can't just get rid of decimal places; you have to account for them in the answer, so the 2.3 must be multiplied by 10^6 to bring it back to the original answer.

The answer to the conversion of 2.3 kg to milligrams is 2.3×10^6 mg.

(b) Change 475 nanograms to milligrams

First change 475 nanograms to micrograms:

$$475\,\text{nanograms} \div 1000 = 0.475\,\text{micrograms}$$

Then change 0.475 micrograms to milligrams:

$$0.475\,\text{micrograms} \div 1000 = 0.000\,475\,\text{mg}$$

This answer in standard form is 4.75×10^{-4}.

The minus power indicates that 4.75 has to be divided to bring it back to the original answer.

LOOK OUT

Full stops and decimal points can be confused. Good practice is to avoid them wherever possible. Use whole numbers and place the unit abbreviation next to the number without leaving a space when you are completing patient records. There are no full stops after the abbreviation.

TIME TO TRY

Convert the following, using standard form if appropriate.

(a) 3420 g to kilograms _____   (b) 0.250 kg to grams _____

(c) 5000 mg to kilograms _____   (d) 1.5 L to millilitres _____

(e) 1 cm to micrometres _____   (f) 550 mL to litres _____

Answers: (a) 3.42 kg (b) 250 g or 2.5×10^2g (c) 0.005 kg or 5.0×10^{-3} kg (d) 1500 mL or 1.5×10^3 mL (e) 10 000 micrometres or 1.0×10^4 micrometres (f) 0.55 L or 5.5×10^{-1} L

If you need some more practice, there are further questions at the end of the chapter.

Where is the mole?

In Table 3.1 the unit that measures the quantity of a substance is called a **mole** (abbreviation, **mol**). It is a more precise measurement than measuring the mass of a substance. You will see it most commonly used in relation to blood chemistry and the administration of some intravenous fluids. You will learn more about moles later in Chapter 5.

$$1 \text{ mole (mol)} = 1000 \text{ millimoles (mmol)}$$

$$1 \text{ millimole (mmol)} = 1000 \text{ micromoles } (\mu\text{mol or mcmol})$$

Change the following.

(a) 1 mole to micromoles _____   (b) 2 millimoles to micromoles _____

Answers: (a) 1.0×10^6 (b) 2.0×10^3.

Don't get hot under the collar

The kelvin is the SI unit for temperature and whilst it is suitable for physicists, it is not user-friendly for clinical practice. The Celsius scale is used in clinical practice and keeps the essence of the SI/metric system.

On this scale 0°C is the freezing point of pure water and 100°C its boiling point. Body temperature is around 37.0°C. You will be glad to hear that you do not need to convert this unit and the only subdivisions are 0.1 of each degree.

RUNNING WORDS

beam balance
gravity
meniscus
millimole (mmol)

mole (mol)
prefix
standard form
surface tension

Système International
d'Unités' (SI units)

Answers to the following questions can be found at the end of the book.

What did you learn?

(a) What is the SI base unit used to measure volume? _____

(b) Name the unit commonly used to measure fluids in clinical practice. _____

(c) You are asked to weigh a baby on a specially modified beam balance. What do you need to know about the equipment before you put the baby on the scales?

_____

(d) What is the name of the line formed by the top of a column of fluid in a container?

_____

(e) A patient drinks six 200 mL glasses of squash during the day. How many litres have been consumed? _____

(f) Which prefix is used for the division of a base unit by 10^{-6}? _____

(g) What is the SI unit used for measuring mass? _____

(h) What is the difference between mass and weight? _____

(i) Change the following to the units indicated.

(i) 250 mg = _____ g

(ii) 1.7 L = _____ mL

(iii) 2 mol = _____ mmol

(iv) 1.33 g = _____ micrograms

(v) 4.3 g = _____ mg

(vi) 250 cm = _____ m

More 'Time to Try' examples

Page 70

Convert the following, using standard form if appropriate.

(a) 2754 g to kilograms _____

(b) 1.43 kg to grams _____

(c) 3500 mg to kilograms _____

(d) 1.2 L to millilitres _____

(e) 1 cm to nanometres _____

(f) 375 mL to litres _____

Web resources

http://www.bnf.org/bnf/bnf/current/104945.htm

The *British National Formulary* gives information about good practices in using abbreviations and SI units. You need to register to access the site, but registration is free. You will find lots of information about medicines, such as doses, side effects, interactions with other drugs and food.

http://www.simetric.co.uk/sibasis.htm

Here you will be able to find out how the SI units are standardised so that a kilogram is a kilogram no matter where it is measured. There are other interesting links to sites expanding on other units as well as other systems of measurement, such as the imperial system which still persists in parts of our lives – do you still buy a pint of milk?

http://www.gcse.com/maths/standard_form.htm

Get some more practice with standard form. Watch out for commas between figures in large numbers. They should not be used in scientific work; figures should be grouped in sets of three, starting from the right, e.g. 2000 *not* 2,000, 12 000 000 *not* 12,000,000, since there can be confusion with decimal points.

http://www.mathsisfun.com/measure/metric-system.html

Some good visual examples of measurement and conversion of units. Beware of American spellings, e.g. me*ter*!

Reference

British Medical Association and Royal Pharmaceutical Society of Great Britain (2008) *British National Formulary*, Number 55. London: British Medical Association and Royal Pharmaceutical Society of Great Britain.

Chapter 4

Drug calculations
Pills, potions and pinpricks

This chapter will help you to prepare for calculating drug doses in clinical practice. It is vital for patient safety and your peace of mind that you are able to give the right drug in the right dose, by the right route, at the right time, to the right patient. Anything less is unacceptable and dangerous. If you have worked through the previous chapters, then this one should present few problems.

When you have completed this chapter, you should be able to:

- Estimate the amount of drug to be given and check that the answer is reasonable.

- Calculate the number of tablets and capsules needed to give the prescribed dose.

- Calculate the amount of liquid medicine needed to give the prescribed dose.

- Calculate the dose based on body weight or body surface area.

- Understand the importance of displacement volume and calculate the volume of drug needed for injection.

Drugs are most commonly given orally but there are other routes that will be discussed in later chapters. Oral medicines can be formulated as capsules, tablets or liquid medicine.

When you have calculated a dose of medication you must first ask yourself if it is a reasonable amount. If you are giving tablets or capsules, calculate again if you are about to give more than four for a single dose. There are some exceptions but they are rare. With liquid medicines, you would not expect to give more than 20 mL as a single dose.

Most tablets and capsules are manufactured in various strengths but may not be in a suitable size for your patient. It is not good practice to cut tablets since it is difficult to be certain that you have the correct dose. The pharmacist will give advice and speak with the prescriber if necessary.

In addition, many tablets and capsules should not be broken because they have a special coating (**enteric coated**) either protecting the drug from being digested too rapidly or to protect the patient's upper digestive tract.

Check that you are in the right lines

Leave the calculator in your pocket. If you have got the last three chapters under your belt then you are well on the way to being competent in using addition, subtraction, multiplication and division. You can use these skills to start your calculation by making a rough estimate of the answer so at least you know that you are on the right lines.

Calculators do have their place but they don't know whether the buttons pressed are the right or wrong ones. Remember RIRO – Rubbish In, Rubbish Out. Relying on a calculator can give you a false sense of security. Calculators are useful for checking your calculation if there a several stages to get the answer.

If you are estimating, the numbers you choose should be ones that are near to the ones in the calculation and easy to calculate in your head. There are no rules for doing this, just what feels comfortable for you, but some suggestions are set out below.

EXAMPLE

Drug quantities are often in decimal fractions. You have seen quite a few examples in Chapter 2 on how to deal with decimal problems.

$$2.7 \times 5.3$$

When you look at these numbers, you can see that they can be rounded to the nearest whole numbers, 3 and 5, so multiply

$$3 \times 5 = 15$$

The actual answer to the sum is 14.31, which is reassuringly close.

4.1 TABLETS, CAPSULES, AND LIQUIDS

The packaging of the drug gives you important information, so become familiar with the layout.

The drug may have two names on the container. One is the name given by the original manufacturer and is known as the **proprietary name**. The name is followed by an ® showing that it is a trademark of the company. The second name, usually in a smaller font, is the **non-proprietary name**. Non-proprietary names are the ones normally used on prescriptions. You may sometimes hear these referred to as generics.

A familiar example is the medicine paracetamol. You can buy a version costing a few pence in any supermarket, but if you choose, you can purchase the original product made by Glaxo Smith Kline which is Panadol®, which costs more. The same difference is seen in branded or non-branded goods that you buy every day.

The other important information is the **drug strength**. Tablets may contain different amounts of the medicine, e.g. ibuprofen can be bought as tablets containing 200 mg of the drug or 400 mg tablets. Make sure that you have the right strength.

> **LOOK OUT**
>
> **Many of the drug manufacturers or packing companies use boxes that all look very similar but contain the same drug of a different strength or a different drug entirely. Double check the labels.**

What is the dose?

Calculation of doses means that we need to use drug names in order to make it more realistic. Don't worry about what the drug does at this point. The 'labels' are not facsimiles, but give you essential information in order to carry out the calculations. This chapter is only about the calculation.

> **KEY POINTS**
>
> The important information that you need for getting to grips with dose calculations:
>
> - The type of **formulation** containing the drug, i.e. tablets, capsules or millilitres of fluid.
> - The amount of drug contained in each tablet, capsule or volume of fluid.

EXAMPLE

Figure 4.1 shows information on labels.

The two labels show the importance of looking at the amount of drug in each capsule. In **Figure 4.1(a)**, there is 250 mg of the antibiotic in each capsule, but in **Figure 4.1(b)** there is twice the dose, 500 mg.

> Amoxil® Capsules 250 mg
> Amoxicillin (as trihydrate)

Figure 4.1(a)

> Amoxil® Capsules 500 mg
> Amoxicillin (as trihydrate)

Figure 4.1(b)

These labels also show how the proprietary and non-proprietary names might appear.

Which is the proprietary name? _____

There is a lot more information on the actual label but we will look at that later.

EXAMPLE 1

A patient is prescribed 500 mg of amoxicillin. How many 250 mg capsules should he been given?

 This is a straightforward example. *You can use your arithmetic skills from the chapter on fractions to solve the problem.*

What you need to find out is how many lots of 250 there are in 500, so 500 has to be divided by 250:

$$\frac{500}{250} = \frac{2}{1} = 2 \text{ capsules}$$

You could probably have done this one in your head but it is not always that simple and you may need to write it down.

The method is the same, but the figures alter depending on the prescription and the strength of the drug involved.

The basic format for this type of calculation is

$$\frac{\text{amount of drug prescribed}}{\text{amount of drug in each tablet/capsule}} = \text{number of tablets/capsules required}$$

APPLYING THE THEORY

Capsules and tablets come from the pharmacy in blister packs or, if the drug is frequently used, like paracetamol, may be dispensed in a plastic screw-top container. The tablets are put into individual disposable containers to give to the patient. You must wash your hands before opening the pack and must not touch the tablet or capsule. Use the lid of the container to select the correct number of tablets.

EXAMPLE 2

Amoxicillin also comes in the form of a liquid medicine, usually for children, but is also suitable for adults who have difficulty with swallowing tablets or capsules.

```
Amoxicillin suspension
125 mg in 5 mL
```

Figure 4.2

The label (**Figure 4.2**) tells you that in every unit, which in this case is 5 mL, there is 125 mg of the drug.

> **LOOK OUT**
>
> **Any liquid medicine needs to be shaken thoroughly to make sure that the drug is evenly distributed, otherwise there may be too much or too little drug in each spoonful.**

EXAMPLE 3

A child is prescribed amoxicillin 250 mg every 6 hours. The liquid medicine is dispensed with the above label. What volume of the medicine should be given?

The child needs 250 mg.

You can use the same method as you used above to begin your calculation:

$$\frac{\text{amount of drug prescribed}}{\text{amount of drug in each unit}}$$

$$\frac{250 \text{ mg}}{125 \text{ mg}} \quad \text{simplifying} = \frac{2}{1} = 2 \quad \text{2 what?}$$

When you simplified fractions in Chapter 2, you divided both the numerator and denominator by the same number: you can also cancel the mg since they are in both the numerator and denominator, leaving you with 2/1. That is, 2 lots of whatever the 125 mg is in. In the last example we needed 2 lots of the capsules to give the dose.

Here, each 125 mg of the drug is contained in 5 mL, so we have to give 2 lots of 5 mL. Thus, 2 × 5 mL = 10 mL, so we need to give 10 mL of the suspension in order to give the prescribed dose of 250 mg.

For liquid medicines, the format that we used for tablets/capsules can be adapted as follows:

$$\frac{\text{amount of drug prescribed}}{\text{amount of drug in each unit}} \times \text{the volume the drug is in (mL)}$$

(the volume is 5 mL in this case)

$$\frac{250 \text{ mg}}{125 \text{ mg}} \times 5 \text{ mL} = \frac{2}{1} \times 5 \text{ mL} = 10 \text{ mL}$$

> **Flucloxacillin syrup**
> **250 mg in 5 mL**

Figure 4.3

EXAMPLE 4

An adult patient has difficulty in swallowing and has been prescribed flucloxacillin syrup 500 mg every 6 hours. How much syrup contains this dose? Use **Figure 4.3** for your calculation.

From the example above

$$\frac{\text{amount of drug prescribed}}{\text{amount of drug in each unit}} \times \text{the volume the drug is in (mL)}$$

$$\frac{500 \text{ mg}}{250 \text{ mg}} \times 5 \text{ mL} = 10 \text{ mL}$$

Look at **Figure 4.4**. Remember to measure at eye level and read the lower line of the meniscus to ensure that the dose is accurate.

> **LOOK OUT**
>
> **A liquid medicine needs to be specifically prescribed, not just substituted for capsules or tablets, even if the dose is the same.**

APPLYING THE THEORY

A liquid medicine that is dispensed as a 5 mL unit is usually measured into a 5 mL measuring spoon and given straight to the patient. Larger volumes which are multiples of 5 mL are dispensed into a graduated measure.

If you have to give a dose that is smaller than 5 mL or the patient has difficulty in taking medicine from a spoon or measure, a disposable **oral syringe** is used.

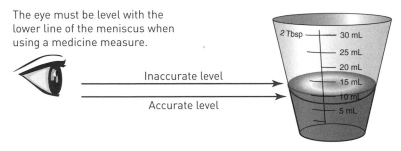

The eye must be level with the lower line of the meniscus when using a medicine measure.

Inaccurate level

Accurate level

2 Tbsp — 30 mL
— 25 mL
— 20 mL
— 15 mL
— 10 mL
— 5 mL

Figure 4.4 Measuring a liquid medicine

Source: Olsen, J. *et al.* (2008) *Medical Dosage Calculations*, Prentice Hall

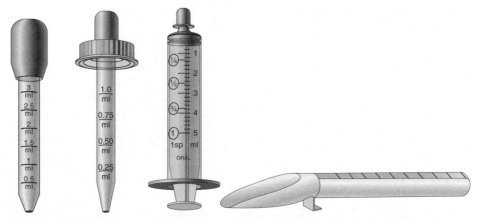

Figure 4.5 Examples of measuring devices used for liquid medicines. The spoon has a hollow, graduated handle for measuring the volume.

Source: Olsen, J. *et al.* (2008) *Medical Dosage Calculations*, Prentice Hall

These are *not* the same as a syringe for injections (which should not be used) and have a cover for the tip (**Figure 4.5**).

Volumes of medicine of less than 1 mL can be given with a graduated dropper.

 Later in the chapter you will be using a similar format for calculating injections, but the unit that the drug for injection is in will vary in volume.

But they're not both milligrams!

Sometimes, the units of the prescribed dose and the units of the drug in the container are not the same.

EXAMPLE 5

Use **Figure 4.6**. A patient is prescribed paracetamol tablets 1 g to be given four times a day. The dose is prescribed in grams and the tablets are 500 mg each.

The first thing you need to do is to change the units so that they are the same. It is best to change the larger to the smaller units rather the other way round. Converting grams to milligrams avoids decimal points.

 Do you remember how to change these units? *Look at Chapter 3 if you need to refresh your memory.*

```
Paracetamol tablets
500 mg
```

Figure 4.6

Convert the dose of 1 g to milligrams:

$$1\,g \times 1000 = 1000\,mg$$

Now you can use the format that you used in Example 1:

$$\frac{\text{amount of drug prescribed}}{\text{amount of drug in each tablet/capsule}} = \text{number of tablets/capsules required}$$

$$\frac{1000\,mg}{500\,mg} = 2\,\text{tablets}$$

Furosemide tablets 20 mg	Simvastatin tablets 10 mg	Amitryptyline solution 25 mg in 5 mL
Carbamazepine tablets 200 mg	Adalat® tablets 5 mg Nifidipine 5 mg	Warfarin tablets 500 micrograms

Figure 4.7

TIME TO TRY

Use the drug labels in **Figure 4.7** to calculate how many tablets or millilitres of liquid medicine a patient should be given for the following prescriptions.

(a) Simvastatin 40 mg _____   (b) Amitryptyline 75 mg _____

(c) Furosemide 40 mg _____   (d) Carbamazepine 1 g _____

(e) Nifidipine 15 mg _____   (f) Warfarin 1 mg _____

(g) Amitryptiline 50 mg _____   (h) Warfarin 1.5 mg _____

Answers: (a) 4 tablets (b) 15 mL (c) 2 tablets (d) 5 tablets (e) 3 tablets (f) 2 tablets (did you remember to change the units to micrograms?) (g) 10 mL (h) 3 tablets

If you need more practice, there are further examples at the end of the chapter.

Compounding the problem

Sometimes two drugs are mixed together in the same tablet. Most of the drugs of this kind have names that start with 'co' indicating that it is a **compound drug**. It is not a popular way of giving drugs as they are in fixed amounts in the one tablet so it is difficult to adjust the dose if needed. It is, however, easier for a patient to take one rather than two tablets.

Examples of these types of drugs are shown on the two labels in **Figure 4.8**.

Co-amoxiclav 250/125 tablets
Amoxicillin 250 mg as trihydrate
Clavulanic acid 125 mg as
potassium salt

Co-codamol 8/500
Codeine phosphate 8 mg
Paracetamol 500 mg

Figure 4.8

These drugs are usually prescribed as 1 or 2 tablets of the compound name, e.g. co-codamol 8/500 tablets every 6 hours, so you do not need to do a calculation, just give the number of tablets prescribed.

LOOK OUT

There may be more than one strength of the compound tablet; for example, co-codamol is also manufactured as co-codamol 15/500 and 30/500.

KEY POINTS

- If in doubt, don't be afraid – ask for help.
- For tablets and capsules use the following format for the calculation:

$$\frac{\text{amount of drug prescribed}}{\text{amount of drug in each tablet/capsule}} = \text{number of tablets/capsules required}$$

- For liquid medicines, use the following format for the calculation:

$$\frac{\text{amount of drug prescribed}}{\text{amount of drug in each unit}} \times \text{the volume the drug is in (mL)}$$

- If the prescribed drug and the dose on the medicine container are in different units, change the larger one to the smaller one to avoid decimal points.

4.2 BODY WEIGHT AND SURFACE AREA

There is always a balance between the benefits of drug therapy and any possible adverse effects that result from treatment. These adverse effects may be relatively minor, such as drowsiness, or they may be life threatening. Sometimes the drug dose has to be tailored to the individual and so it is calculated according to the patient's weight or **body surface area**. This is particularly true for children.

Body weight

You may already be familiar with this type of calculation if you have a pet dog or cat. If it needs worm tablets, then you have to weigh it and give a number of tablets according to its weight.

A patient's weight needs to be recorded accurately before the drug is first given and checked at least weekly during treatment.

APPLYING THE THEORY

One of the most common drug groups given as mg/kg body weight is that used to treat cancers – cytotoxic drugs. Many patients with these diseases lose weight rapidly, so what is a suitable dose at the start of treatment may be too much three or four weeks later and may need adjustment.

EXAMPLE 6

A male patient weighs 72 kg and is prescribed a drug (doesn't matter what at this stage) which is to be given in a dose of 4 mg per kilogram of body weight – usually written as 4 mg/kg.

The two pieces of information that you need to work out the dose are the amount of drug per kilogram and the patient's body weight.

For every kilogram that the patient weighs, he is given 4 mg of the drug, so in this case 72 is multiplied by 4 to find out the total number of milligrams he has to be given:

$$\text{body weight (kg)} \times \text{amount of drug per kg} = \text{dose required}$$
$$72 \qquad \times \qquad 4 \text{ mg} \qquad = 288 \text{ mg}$$

 This is the same principle as we used in Chapter 1 for multiplying numbers together.

Body surface area (BSA)

The skin is the largest of our body organs and has the ability to stretch to accommodate the body mass of the growing child or adults who are growing out rather than up. Surface area increases with body height and weight. Skin surface area is measured in metres squared. An adult who is 1.70 m tall and weighs 65 kg has a surface area of 1.8 m^2. It is a good indicator of an individual's metabolic state.

There are several formulae for working out BSA but you really wouldn't want to try them! The easy way to solve the problem is to use a prepared chart called a **nomogram** (see Appendix I).

The dose prescribed for a patient whose BSA is 1.75 m^2 is 300 mg per m^2.

The formula for this calculation is

$$\text{BSA} \times \text{dose per m}^2 = \text{dose required}$$
$$1.75 \times \quad 300 \text{ mg} \quad = 525 \text{ mg}$$

TIME TO TRY

1. (a) Calculate the dose of the drug to be given if a patient weighing 60 kg is prescribed a dose of 6 mg/kg. _____

   (b) Calculate the dose of the drug to be given if a patient weighing 73 kg is prescribed a dose of 3 mg/kg. _____

   (c) Calculate the dose of the drug to be given if a patient weighing 70 kg is prescribed a dose of 450 micrograms/kg (give your answer in mg). _____

(d) Calculate the dose of the drug to be given if a patient weighing 66 kg is prescribed a dose of 15 mg/kg. _____

2. (a) Calculate the dose of the drug to be given if a patient with a surface area of 1.75 m^2 is prescribed a dose of 500 mg/m^2. _____

(b) Calculate the dose of the drug to be given if a patient with a surface area of 1.55 m^2 is prescribed a dose of 250 mg/m^2. _____

(c) Calculate the dose of the drug to be given if a patient with a surface area of 1.69 m^2 is prescribed a dose of 300 mg/m^2. _____

(d) Calculate the dose of the drug to be given if a patient with a surface area of 1.88 m^2 is prescribed a dose of 250 mg/m^2. _____

Answers: **1.** (a) 360 mg (b) 219 mg (c) 31.5 mg (d) 990 mg   **2.** (a) 875 mg (b) 387.5 mg (c) 507 mg (d) 470 mg

If you need more practice, there are further examples at the end of the chapter.

So what?

Finding the dose according to body weight or surface area is not usually an end in itself – you still have to calculate the dose from the actual drug strength.

Quite often, the dose that you have calculated from the mg/kg or mg/m^2 is the total amount of the drug that the patient will need for the whole day (**total daily dose, TDD**).

Many medicines are given three times a day or every 4 hours, so the dose you have calculated will need to be divided into smaller doses, given over the whole 24 hours as prescribed.

EXAMPLE 7

A patient is prescribed 20 mg/kg body weight. The patient weighs 70 kg, so the total dose is

$$70 \times 20 \text{ mg} = 1400 \text{ mg}$$

The prescription states that the total daily dose is to be given in equal doses every 6 hours.

You now have to divide 1400 mg by the number of doses to be given in 24 hours.

The prescription doesn't actually tell you how many times a day, but every 6 hours gives you a clue:

$$\frac{24 \text{ hours}}{6 \text{ hours}} = 4 \text{ times a day}$$

The next step is to divide the total daily dose by 4 to find the quantity of a single dose:

$$\text{Single dose} = \frac{1400 \text{ mg}}{4} = 350 \text{ mg}$$

83

EXAMPLE 8

A patient is prescribed 5 mg/kg body weight. The patient weighs 65 kg so the total daily dose is

$$65 \times 5\,mg = 325\,mg$$

The prescription states that the dose is to be given three times a day. This is *not* the same as Example 7. This time, 325 mg is not to be divided but given three times during the day.

LOOK OUT

Read the instructions carefully when you have to calculate doses involving body weight or surface area. Make sure that you check how the result is to be used. Three times a day is not the same as divided into three equal doses.

APPLYING THE THEORY

Children's drug doses are often prescribed as a total daily dose, based on surface area, which is divided into a number of single doses spread throughout the day.

KEY POINTS

- Use a nomogram to find body surface area.
- Weigh patients regularly to ensure correct dose is given.
- Check whether doses are three times a day or divided into three doses.

TIME TO TRY

(a) Calculate the quantity of a single dose of a drug to be given if a patient with a surface area of 1.8 m^2 is prescribed a dose of 100 mg/m^2 to be given divided into four doses. _____

(b) Calculate the quantity of a single dose of a drug to be given if a patient with a body weight of 78 kg is prescribed 4 mg/kg to be given in divided doses every 6 hours. _____

(c) Calculate the quantity of a drug to be given if a patient with a surface area of 1.74 m^2 is prescribed a dose of 150 mg/m^2 to be given three times a day.

(d) Calculate the quantity of a single dose of a drug to be given if a patient with a body weight of 66 kg is prescribed 5 mg/kg to be given in divided doses every 4 hours. _____

Answers: (a) 45 mg (b) 78 mg (c) 261 mg (d) 55 mg

If you need more practice, there are further examples at the end of the chapter.

4.3 INJECTIONS

You have covered quite a lot of different types of drug calculations, all of which are for oral medications. This is sometimes called the **enteral** route.

When patients are unable to swallow or the drug is destroyed by the chemicals in the intestine, medication is given by the **parenteral** route: an injection with a hypodermic syringe and needle. The manufacturers put the drug in sterile glass or plastic containers called **ampoules** or a **vial** with a 'rubber' stopper (**Figure 4.9**).

The drug may already be in a solution but may also come as a powder to which sterile liquid must be added and then shaken to make it dissolve.

Most drugs given by injection are measured in grams or fractions of a gram, but some are measured not by the weight of the drug but by the drug's biological activity and are measured in units. Units in this context must be written in *full* to avoid confusion with m and n. *These units will be discussed in Chapter 5.*

For the time being it is most useful first to get to grips with the injection of drugs that are measured in SI units.

Surface tension causes miniscule droplets of liquid to stick to the sides of a container, so allowance is made to ensure that a full dose can be removed. It is important that the calculated dose is measured carefully, and you do not just take every last drop out of the ampoule.

Powder takes up space in the mixture so must be taken into account when making up the final volume. This is called the **displacement value**. Some drugs dissolve so well that the space occupied makes no significant difference to the final volume. Check the box insert to confirm the type and volume of fluid needed to mix with the drug, taking into account any displacement value. Most of the time sterile water is used, but occasionally 0.9% sodium chloride or another fluid may be used.

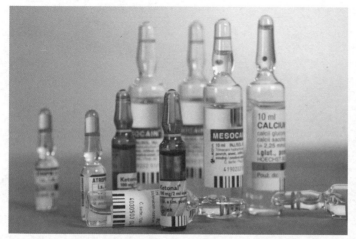
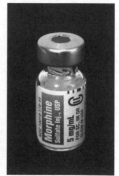

Figure 4.9 Examples of glass ampoules and vials with a rubber stopper
Source: Profimedia International s.r.o./Alamy (l); Scott Camazine/Science Photo Library (r)

> **LOOK OUT**
> Ignoring the displacement value will result in a drug error.

Choose your tools

Your choice of syringe will depend on the volume of fluid you need to draw up for the final dose. It is best to use the smallest syringe that will hold volume you need. There is always a drop of fluid left at the tip of the syringe. This is called the **dead space** and is allowed for in the calibration of the syringe.

Different-sized syringes have different levels of accuracy in their **calibrations** (**Figure 4.10**): 1 mL syringes have divisions of 0.01 mL, so you can measure accurately to two decimal places – they are used when the volume to be given is less than 1 mL and are particularly useful for paediatric doses; 2 mL syringes have

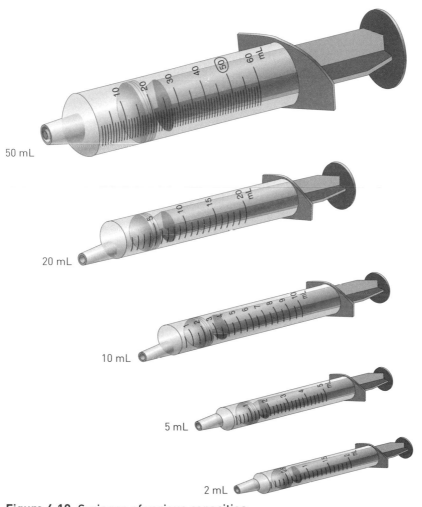

Figure 4.10 Syringes of various capacities

Source: Olsen, J. *et al.* (2008) *Medical Dosage Calculations*, Prentice Hall

0.1 mL divisions, 5 mL syringes have 0.2 mL divisions, and 10 and 20 mL syringes have 1 mL divisions.

EXAMPLE 9

The example in **Figure 4.11(a)** identifies that the final volume is 10 mL, and contains 500 mg of amoxicillin.

This means that 1 mL contains 50 mg (500 mg/10 mL = 50 mg/mL).

The displacement volume is 0.4 mL. If you add 10 mL of diluting fluid, the reconstituted volume will be 10.4 mL.

There are now 48 mg/mL not 50 mg/mL (500 mg/10.4 = 48 mg/mL). If the prescription required 250 mg and you drew up 5 mL of this solution, the patient would receive 240 mg instead (5 × 48 mg = 240 mg).

To get the correct dilution, you need to add 10 mL − 0.4 mL = 9.6 mL.

If you put in 10 mL of diluent and use the whole 500 mg, the 10.4 mL may not fit in the 10 mL syringe!

APPLYING THE THEORY

It is essential in practice to follow the drug manufacturers' instructions regarding the reconstitution, administration and storage of drugs for injection. These are usually found on the package insert.

> ### LOOK OUT
>
> The instructions may be different depending on whether the drug is to be given as an intramuscular or intravenous injection. Make sure that you read the correct information on the **summary of product characteristics** sheet (also known as a data sheet) which is a more detailed than the package insert.

Use Figure 4.11(a) to calculate the volume of drug you need to draw up into a syringe in order to give a patient 250 mg of amoxicillin by injection. Use the format that you used for liquid medicines – it works just the same here:

$$\frac{\text{amount of drug prescribed}}{\text{amount of drug in each unit}} \times \text{the volume the drug is in (mL)}$$

$$\frac{250 \text{ mg}^1}{500 \text{ mg}^{2\ 1}} \times 10^5 \text{ mL} = 5 \text{ mL}$$

> Amoxil® injection
> Amoxicillin 500 mg as
> sodium salt when
> reconstituted to 10 mL
> to give 50 mg/mL
> Displacement volume 0.4 mL

Figure 4.11(a)

> Diazepam injection solution
> 5 mg/mL

Figure 4.11(b)

You can do a quick rough check for this one. If you recognised that 250 is half of 500, then it would follow that you need half of the volume of the contents. This is half of 10 mL so the answer is 5 mL – not too tough was it?

Keep this simple calculation in mind if you don't like the look of a calculation with what you might think are difficult numbers. They are all done in the same way so there is no need to get worried.

Use **Figure 4.11(b)** to calculate the volume of solution needed to give an intra-muscular injection of 3 mg of diazepam:

$$\frac{\text{amount of drug prescribed}}{\text{amount of drug in each unit}} \times \text{the volume the drug is in (mL)}$$

$$\frac{3 \text{ mg}}{5 \text{ mg}} \times 1 \text{ mL} = 0.6 \text{ mL}$$

Which size of syringe would you use to draw up this volume of fluid?

A 1 mL syringe would give you the best level of accuracy. In general, smaller syringes are cheaper, so this is another reason for choosing the smallest that will accommodate the volume needed.

TIME TO TRY

Use the drug labels in **Figure 4.12** to carry out the following calculations.

What volume of fluid do you need for the following injections?

You may need to correct your answer to one decimal place unless the volume is less than 1 mL, in which case it is two places, due to the limitations of the syringes.

(a) dexamethasone 800 micrograms _____

(b) furosemide 10 mg _____

(c) metoclopramide 10 mg _____

(d) adrenaline 500 micrograms _____

Metoclopramide injection 5 mg/mL	Flucloxacillin injection Powder for reconstitution 250 mg/5 mL Displacement volume 0.2 mL	Crystapen® injection Benzylpenicillin sodium Powder for reconstitution 600 mg/5 mL Displacement volume 0.4 mL
Dexamethasone injection 4 mg/mL	Furosemide injection 20 mg/2 mL	Adrenaline (epinephrine) injection 1 mg/mL

Figure 4.12

How much sterile water needs to be added to the following in order to reconstitute them to produce the correct strength of solution?

(e) flucloxacillin injection _____   (f) benzylpenicillin _____

Following reconstitution, what volume do you need for the following injections?

(g) flucloxacillin 125 mg _____   (h) benzylpenicillin 450 mg _____

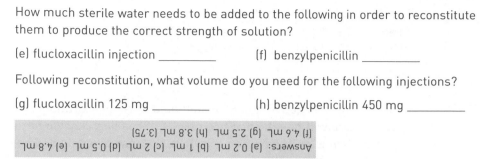

Answers: (a) 0.2 mL (b) 1 mL (c) 2 mL (d) 0.5 mL (e) 4.8 mL (f) 4.6 mL (g) 2.5 mL (h) 3.8 mL (3.75)

If you need more practice, there are further examples at the end of the chapter.

Drawing up the dose

Now that you have cracked the calculation of the volume of drug that is needed to give the correct dose, all you have to do is to get the correct measurement into the syringe.

It is not the purpose of this chapter, or any other in this book, to go into discussions about needle size, changing of needles, aseptic technique or injection sites. Views on these topics will vary with the latest evidence-based practice, so we will look at the mechanics of getting the right dose into the syringe.

Bits and pieces

The syringe is made up of:

● The barrel, which is hollow and has the calibrations marked on the outer surface.

● The plunger, which fits snugly into the barrel and has a rubber tip with a top and bottom ring. It can be pulled to suck fluid into the barrel and pushed to expel the fluid.

● The tip, for attachment to the hub of the needle. This may be a simple push-fit tip but for a more secure attachment may be a twist mechanism known as a **Luer-lock**. **Figure 4.13** shows a push-fit syringe.

APPLYING THE THEORY

There are other types of syringes that you will encounter in practice, each with its own special functions and uses. You will find some that come complete with

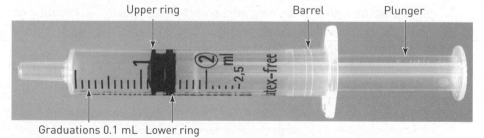

Upper ring   Barrel   Plunger

Graduations 0.1 mL   Lower ring

Figure 4.13 A 2.5 mL syringe with a push-fit tip

Source: Wellcome Images

needles, others with special devices such as retractable needles or finger guards. Specialised syringes are more expensive than the standard syringe, so you must choose the right one for the job in hand.

> **LOOK OUT**
>
> Do not use injection syringes to administer oral preparations. Oral syringes cannot be attached to a needle. It has been known for an oral preparation to be given as an injection, because a needle had been attached to an injection syringe to withdraw the medicine from a bottle. The patient suffered severe tissue damage.

Ready to measure?

Figure 4.13 is a diagram of a syringe containing fluid. The plunger has been pulled back and a measured amount of medication has been drawn into the syringe. The graduations are 0.1 mL and the reading of volume is taken at the level of the upper ring. In this case the volume of fluid is over the 1 mL mark and two graduations more. This makes this particular volume of fluid 1.2 mL.

One of the problems that you will encounter when drawing up fluid into a syringe is that air bubbles may get in. This will affect the accuracy of the measurement and need to be removed. You will meet exceptions to having a bubble in the syringe with drugs that come already prepared in a syringe.

APPLYING THE THEORY

Drawing up a specific amount of fluid into a syringe is a skill that needs practice. Drugs are expensive, so get your technique right by practising with clean equipment and tap water. You will need to practise removing air bubbles and no doubt you will find the way that suits you best.

> **LOOK OUT**
>
> Expelling air from an injection syringe needs to be done with care because it is difficult to get rid of the air without losing some of the drug in the form of almost invisible droplets. This could mean that you could get them on your skin or inhale particles of the drug. The mist can spread throughout the environment and if an antibiotic may contribute to organisms becoming resistant to the antibiotic.

TIME TO TRY

What is the volume of drug in the syringes in **Figures 4.14(a)** and **(b)**? Remember to take the reading at the level of the upper ring of the plunger.

Answers: **4.14(a)** 4.2 mL **4.14(b)** 5.0 mL

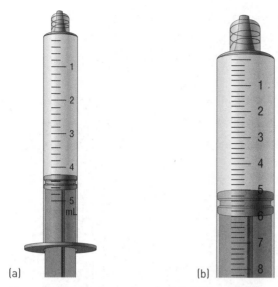

Figure 4.14 Measurement of fluid in syringes

RUNNING WORDS

ampoule	enteral	oral syringe
body surface area	enteric coated	parenteral
calibration	formulation	proprietary name
compound drug	generics	summary of product
dead space	Luer-lock	characteristics
displacement value	nomogram	total daily dose (TTD)
drug strength	non-proprietary name	vial

Answers to the following questions can be found at the end of the book.

What did you learn?

(a) Make a rough estimate for the following calculation: $4.9 \times 3.2 = $ _____

(b) What is the actual answer to the above? _____

(c) What is the proprietary name for a drug? _____

(d) How should the level of liquid medicine be checked when using a medicine measure? _____

(e) What container should be used to measure a dose of 0.3 mL of a liquid medicine?

_____

91

(f) Which two body measurements can be used to get a more individualised dose of medicine? _____

(g) Calculate the total daily dose for a patient who has a body weight of 62 kg and is to receive 3 mg/kg/day. _____

(h) Calculate the number of tablets or millilitres of liquid of drug needed for the following prescriptions using **Figure 4.15**.

   (i) Furosemide 30 mg _____   (ii) Warfarin 1.5 mg _____

   (iii) Nifidipine 10 mg _____   (iv) Amoxicillin 125 mg _____

   (v) Prednisolone 10 mg _____   (vi) Flucloxacillin 250 mg _____

Warfarin tablets 500 micrograms	Adalat® tablets 5 mg Nifidipine 5 mg	Flucloxacillin syrup 250 mg in 5 mL
Furosemide injection 20 mg/2 mL	Amoxicillin injection Powder for reconstitution 250 mg/5 mL Displacement volume 0.2 mL	Prednisolone tablets 2.5 mg

Figure 4.15

More 'Time to Try' examples

Page 80

Use the drug labels in **Figure 4.16** to calculate how many tablets or millilitres of liquid medicine a patient should be given for the following prescriptions.

(a) Atenolol 50 mg _____

(b) Cimetidine 100 mg _____

Atenolol tablets 25 mg	Digoxin tablets 62.5 micrograms	Cimetidine solution 200 mg in 5 mL
Salbutamol tablets 2 mg	Emtriva® solution 10 mg in 1 mL Emtricitabine	Prednisolone tablets 2.5 mg

Figure 4.16

(c) Digoxin 125 micrograms _____

(d) Salbutamol 4 mg _____

(e) Emtricitabine 150 mg _____

(f) Prednisolone 7.5 mg _____

(g) Cimetidine 300 mg _____

(h) Emtricitabine 120 mg _____

Page 82-3

1. (a) Calculate the dose of the drug to be given if a patient weighing 80 kg is prescribed a dose of 4 mg/kg. _____

(b) Calculate the dose of the drug to be given if a patient weighing 63 kg is prescribed a dose of 5 mg/kg. _____

(c) Calculate the dose of the drug to be given if a patient weighing 70 kg is prescribed a dose of 200 micrograms/kg (give your answer in mg). _____

(d) Calculate the dose of the drug to be given if a patient weighing 77 kg is prescribed a dose of 10 mg/kg. _____

2. (a) Calculate the dose of the drug to be given if a patient with a surface area of 1.85 m^2 is prescribed a dose of 250 mg/m^2. _____

(b) Calculate the dose of the drug to be given if a patient with a surface area of 1.65 m^2 is prescribed a dose of 50 mg/ m^2. _____

(c) Calculate the dose of the drug to be given if a patient with a surface area of 1.75 m^2 is prescribed a dose of 200 mg/m^2. _____

(d) Calculate the dose of the drug to be given if a patient with a surface area of 1.90 m^2 is prescribed a dose of 150 mg/m^2. _____

Page 84

(a) Calculate the quantity of a single dose of a drug to be given if a patient with a surface area of 1.89 m^2 is prescribed a dose of 2 mg/m^2 to be given divided into three doses. _____

(b) Calculate the quantity of a single dose of a drug to be given if a patient with a body weight of 64 kg is prescribed 3 mg/kg to be given divided into four equal doses. _____

(c) Calculate the quantity of a drug to be given if a patient with a surface area of 1.7 m^2 is prescribed a dose of 200 mg/m^2 to be given three times a day. _____

(d) Calculate the quantity of a single dose of a drug to be given if a patient with a body weight of 60 kg is prescribed 8 mg/kg to be given in divided doses every 4 hours. _____

Metoclopramide injection 5 mg/mL	Cefotaxime injection Powder for reconstitution 500 mg/2 mL Displacement volume 0.2 mL	Rochephin® injection Ceftriaxone as sodium salt Powder for reconstitution 500 mg/5 mL Displacement volume 0.4 mL
Dexamethasone injection 4 mg/mL	Furosemide injection 20 mg/2 mL	Adrenaline (epinephrine) injection 1 mg/mL

Figure 4.17

Page 88

Use the drug labels in **Figure 4.17** to carrying out the following calculations.

What volume of fluid do you need for the following injections?

(a) Dexamethasone 1 mg _____   (b) Furosemide 15 mg _____

(c) Metoclopramide 7.5 mg _____   (d) Adrenaline 250 micrograms _____

How much sterile water needs to be added to the following in order to reconstitute them to produce the correct strength of solution?

(e) Cefotaxime injection _____   (f) Ceftriaxone _____

Following reconstitution, what volume do you need for the following injections?

(g) Cefotaxime 200 mg _____   (h) Ceftriaxone 350 mg _____

Web resources

http://www.google.co.uk/search?sourceid=navclient&ie=UTF-8&rlz=1T4HPEB_en___GB207&q=summary+of+product+characteristics
This link gives you an insight into how EU regulations govern the production of drugs and the summary of product characteristics that drug manufacturers need to provide for users of the product.

http://www.halls.md/body-surface-area/refs.htm
A number of formulae are given for calculating surface area – just for interest!

http://www.medicines.org.uk/medguides.aspx
When you visit this site, click on 'visit medicines guide', then on 'browse medicines' on the left menu. You will then have an A–Z to find the drug you want. You will find links for patient information and the Specific Product Information.

http://www.bioscience.org/atlases/clinical/nomogram/nomoadul.htm
A nonogram for body surface area for adults.

http://cmbi.bjmu.cn/servese/clinical/nomogram/nomochil.htm
A nomogram for body surface area for children.

Chapter 5

Drug concentrations
The jokers in the pack

In Chapter 4, you used the commonest types of calculations that you will encounter in practice. Special drugs need special equipment so you need to be sure that you use the right tools for the right job. Although diabetes is a common condition, most sufferers manage their own drug therapy, so you will need to teach them how to administer their medication.

When you have completed this chapter, you should be able to:

- Name drugs that are normally prescribed in units.
- Demonstrate how to measure drugs that are to be given as units.
- Define moles and millimoles and how they equate with other SI units.

5.1 DRUGS MEASURED IN UNITS

Some drugs are produced from animal sources or from **synthetic** variations of these products. The drugs are measured in **units**/mL of activity rather than milligrams, so the calculation is slightly different from the usual format.

You have probably come across units on the labels of food packets, where vitamins are listed in units. Each substance has an agreed international standard for the value of its unit which reflects the expected activity of the substance in the body.

One of the commonest substances measured in units in clinical practice is **insulin**, which is used in the management of diabetes mellitus, a condition where the blood glucose is not well controlled.

There are others, but as you will see there is no overall value for a unit, just a standard for each substance.

EXAMPLES: 1 unit represents

45.5 micrograms of a standard preparation of insulin
0.6 micrograms of a standard preparation of penicillin
0.2 micrograms of a standard preparation of tuberculin
50 micrograms of vitamin C

Insulin

The calculation of the dose of insulin is very straightforward. It comes in multi-dose vials that all contain 100 units/mL. Special insulin syringes are used which are graduated in units rather than millilitres (**Figure 5.1**). The standard **insulin syringe** is calibrated in 2 unit divisions up to 100 units. Patients may need a small dose (less than 50 units) and so there are low-dose syringes graduated in 1 unit divisions up to 50 units.

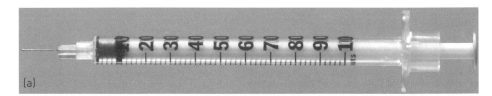

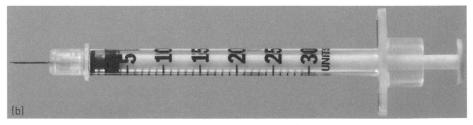

Figure 5.1 Insulin syringes: (a) 100 unit syringe; (b) 30 unit syringe

Source: Wellcome Images

The drug is prescribed in units so what you need to draw up is the correct dose in units in the special syringe. It is best to use the smallest syringe for the volume needed as you get a better degree of accuracy.

For ease of administration, patients may be prescribed their insulin in the form of cartridges that are administered with a pen device. One press of the pen will deliver 2 units of insulin or it can be preset to deliver a fixed number of units, which is useful for people with poor eyesight or reduced manual dexterity.

> **LOOK OUT**
> The word unit must be written in full and is not abbreviated.

Sources of insulin

Although we talk about insulin as if it were a single item, in reality there are many very different products. It is beyond the scope of this book to go into any depth about the different types but you should be aware of the main potential problems.

Insulin was originally an extract of pig pancreas or less commonly of bovine pancreas. So-called human insulin is not an extract but is made in the laboratory by combining the human gene which codes for insulin with the genetic material of bacteria or yeasts. The label on the vial of this type of insulin shows its origin by the letters rDNA, an abbreviation for **recombinant Deoxyribose Nucleic Acid**.

You need to make sure that the patient is aware of the source of their insulin as they may have religious objections to some types.

These different sources of insulin are further refined so that they work over different periods of time. See **Table 5.1**.

Table 5.1 Types of insulin

Approximate length of action	Type of insulin	Examples
Short acting Onset within 1/2 to 1 hour Peak effect 3–4 hours Lasts no more than 8 hours	Soluble Human insulin analogues	Actrapid® Humulin S® NovoRapid® Humalog®
Intermediate acting Onset within 1–2 hours Peak effect 4–12 hours Lasts 12–24 hours	Isophane Insulin zinc suspension	Insulatard® Humulin I® Monotard® Ultratard®
Long acting Onset within 1–3 hours No peak Lasts 24–36 hours	Insulin zinc suspension (crystalline) Insulin glarine	Ultratard® Lantus®

APPLYING THE THEORY

Every patient has their dose of insulin tailored to their needs, using particular combinations of insulin at different times of the day. The patient needs to learn to manage their condition independently as soon as possible and should be involved in the drawing up and checking of the insulin dose.

LOOK OUT

Insulin syringes must not be used for any other drug that is measured in units.

TIME TO TRY

How much insulin is in the following syringes if it is drawn up to the level of the arrow?

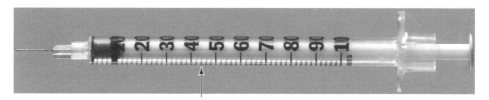

(a)

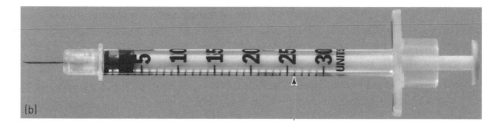

(b)

Answers: (a) 44 units (b) 26 units.

As you have seen from Table 5.1, different types of insulin have different lengths of activity. Rather than giving injections every 3 or 4 hours to cover the 24-hour period, short-acting insulin can be combined with a longer acting type to cover a longer period.

The insulin can be ready mixed as **biphasic** insulin or it can be mixed using some of each type in a standard insulin syringe. Each type of insulin needs to be prescribed separately and drawn up into the syringe with care.

Always draw up the units of soluble insulin first, then the long-acting insulin. If you accidentally draw up the incorrect amount of the long-acting insulin, then you will need to discard the whole syringe and start again.

Wherever possible, the patient should be prescribed the ready-mixed biphasic type.

LOOK OUT

It is important that when different types of insulin are mixed, they are both from the same source.

One brand of insulin must not be substituted for another of a similar type since each patient is stabilised on a particular brand and combination of insulin and changing the regime can lead to uncontrolled glucose levels.

KEY POINTS

- Insulin is measured in units.
- Insulin syringes are graduated in units and are only used for insulin.
- Insulin can be extracted from pig or cow pancreas or from synthetic human insulin.
- Short-acting insulin should be drawn up into the syringe before the long-acting type.
- One source of insulin must not be substituted for another.

Heparin (unfractionated heparin)

Many patients have problems with their blood clotting too easily or develop clots as a result of prolonged periods of immobility such as complex surgery, fractures or sitting for a long time in aeroplanes.

Clots in the circulation can be life threatening, so patients at risk of developing a thrombosis (clot) may be given the **anticoagulant** heparin sodium as a subcutaneous injection every 8–12 hours, either to prevent or treat clot formation.

Initial treatment of a blood clot may include intravenous **heparin** given via a syringe pump. *See Chapter 7 for more details about this equipment.*

Like insulin, heparin is prescribed in units. Heparin is not drawn up in special syringes and is available in single and multi-dose vials. There is a wide range of doses prescribed, depending on the patient's weight, medical condition and blood results.

The strengths of heparin available are as follows:

1000 units/mL	in ampoules of	1 mL, 5 mL, 10 mL, 20 mL
	and vials of	5 mL
5000 units/mL	in ampoules of	1 mL, 5 mL
	and vials of	5 mL
25 000 units/mL	in ampoules of	1 mL
	and vials of	5 mL

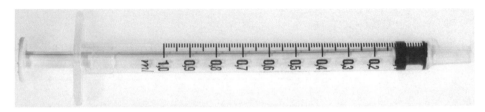

Figure 5.2 A 1 mL syringe with divisions of 0.01 mL

Source: Wellcome Images

Small doses of heparin need to be drawn up into a 1 mL syringe (**Figure 5.2**). These are often needed for paediatric doses.

Heparin is also produced in pre-filled syringes, again coming in several strengths.

You do not need to remember all the different strengths of heparin but you need to appreciate the number of different preparations and the potential for error. You will need to choose the most appropriate concentration taking into account the amount prescribed and the comfort of the patient.

APPLYING THE THEORY

Giving anticoagulants is only part of the prevention of the development of blood clots, particularly in the deep veins of the legs. Everyone should be aware of the advice given to passengers flying long distance: keep hydrated, move legs as much as possible, breathe deeply and wear support socks. This advice is also appropriate for patients in hospital.

Calculating the dose of heparin

These calculations are carried out in the same way as other types of calculation except that the strength is in units per millilitre rather than milligrams per millilitre.

EXAMPLE

A patient is prescribed 15 000 units of heparin to be given by subcutaneous injection every 12 hours. Calculate the smallest volume required to give the dose.

If you use 5000 units/mL you will need

$$\frac{^3\cancel{15\,000\text{ units}}}{^1\cancel{5000\text{ units}}} \times 1 \text{ mL} = 3 \text{ mL}$$

This is quite a large volume for subcutaneous injection, which could be painful for the patient. If you use 25 000 units/mL then you will need

$$\frac{^3\cancel{15\,000\text{ units}}}{^5\cancel{25\,000\text{ units}}} \times 1 \text{ mL} = \frac{3}{5} \text{ mL} = \frac{6}{10} = 0.6 \text{ mL}$$

This volume is less than 1 mL, so should be drawn up into a 1 mL syringe to get an accurate reading. The syringe is graduated in 1/10 mL so you need to change 3/5 to the equivalent fraction 6/10 (0.6 mL) to measure the dose accurately.

TIME TO TRY

Calculate the following doses of heparin for subcutaneous injection, giving the smallest volume.

(a) 25 000 units _____   (b) 5000 units _____   (c) 2500 units _____

(d) 8000 units _____   (e) 10 000 units _____   (f) 4500 units _____

Answers: (a) 1 mL of 25 000 units/mL (b) 1 mL of 5000 units/mL (c) 0.5 mL of 5000 units/mL (d) 1.6 mL of 5000 units/mL (e) 0.4 mL of 25 000 units/mL (f) 0.9 mL of 5000 units/mL.

If you need more practice, there are further examples at the end of the chapter.

LOOK OUT

The whole point of giving heparin is to reduce clot formation in the blood, but there is always a possibility of overdoing things and causing bleeding. Patients' blood should be tested on a daily basis. You will learn more about monitoring the effects of heparin in pharmacology sessions.

If you are giving patients medication, then you are also responsible for monitoring the effects. You should observe your patient for signs of bleeding from the gums, bruising (**contusion**), nose bleeds (**epistaxis**) or traces of blood in the urine (**haematuria**). Any of these should be reported to the doctor immediately.

Low-molecular-weight heparin (LMWH)

As the name suggests, these heparins differ from **unfractionated** heparin in the size and weight of the molecules. This affects the way in which the drug is used by the body as well as its anticoagulant properties. LMWHs are mainly given in the prevention (prophylaxis) of thrombosis but some may be used in the treatment of conditions such as deep-vein thrombosis.

Advantages of **LMWHs**:

● Longer duration of action, so need to be given only once daily.

● Can be tailored more closely to the individual by prescribing according to body weight.

● Do not need such close laboratory monitoring.

Doses may be prescribed in milligrams per kg of body in treatment regimes or as a standard dose in **prophylaxis**.

There are a number of LMWH products all of which are packaged in pre-filled syringes of various doses as well as multi-dose vials.

> **LOOK OUT**
>
> Make sure that you have the correct strength in the syringe since there may be as many as seven different strength pre-filled syringes of any one product.
>
> You must be clear about the dose prescribed. Some prescribers will state the dose in units, others in units per kg or yet others in millilitres of a particular strength solution. If in doubt, don't give it – CHECK.

Revisit Chapter 4 on calculating drug doses using body weight, since these LMWHs may be prescribed per kg of body weight.

KEY POINTS

- Unfractionated heparin ampoules contain different strengths so care must be taken to ensure that the correct dose is given.
- Patients must be monitored for signs of overdose.
- LMWH is given per kg of body weight, so accurate weighing of the patient is vital.

APPLYING THE THEORY

Pre-filled syringes have very small needles and the injections are given at right angles to the skin. There is a bubble of air in these syringes but you do not need to expel it before giving the drug.

5.2 MEASURING IN MOLES

As cute as they are, the little furry chaps have nothing to do with biochemistry.

In the last chapter, the **mole** kept a low profile, except for some basic changing of units, which was just like changing any other units in SI.

In practice, most of the occasions where you will come across the mole will be in the reports on a patient's blood biochemistry where many tests such as blood glucose, sodium, potassium and other blood **electrolytes** are measured in millimoles or micromoles per litre of blood.

Whilst you will not normally be required to work out these concentrations, the next part of the chapter gives you an understanding of the units used for these measurements.

APPLYING THE THEORY

Many patients need fluid replacement therapy if they are dehydrated or have had a fluid loss as a result of surgery. It is important that the normal levels of electrolytes are maintained. Fluids are given through a vein (intravenously) and contain electrolytes that are measured in millimoles, usually at a similar concentration as in the blood. You need to be able to check the fluid concentrations against the prescription.

It is important to have a basic understanding of the moles and fractions of moles used to measure concentrations of substances in the body in order to be aware of when there are deviations from normal.

We need to start with some easy chemistry. You do not need to be a brain surgeon or a rocket scientist to have a grasp of the subject, but you do need to have a good imagination of how small things can get.

Everything is made up of very small particles called **atoms**. **Elements** are pure substances that are made up of atoms of all the same kind. Are you still with me?

Look at an example that is probably familiar to you – water. What is the chemical formula for water? _____

H_2O is the chemical formula for water. This is a molecule of water, which in turn is made up of the basic particles, or elements hydrogen (H) and oxygen (O). The **formula** tells us that there are two atoms of hydrogen and one of oxygen. Atoms are very small – you can't see them; you have to take it on trust.

Every element has its own particular **relative atomic mass** (weight). Here are a few examples of elements used in clinical practice:

carbon	(C)	12
hydrogen	(H)	1
oxygen	(O)	16
potassium	(K)	39
sodium	(Na)	23
chlorine	(Cl)	35.5

(There is a fuller list in Appendix C.)

If you had enough atoms or molecules of an element or compound, you could weigh them in grams or milligrams.

Carbon is used as the standard for measuring a mole. A mole is the relative atomic mass of a substance in grams; 12 g of carbon is a mole of carbon, which is its relative atomic mass in grams.

It follows that a mole of chlorine has a mass of 35.5 g and that of potassium, 39 g. You can also have a mole of a compound such as sodium chloride (NaCl), better known as the salt that you sprinkle on your chips.

If we take the relative atomic mass of each of the components, then we have

Na 23 + Cl 35.5

If these two relative atomic masses are added, we find that the total is 58.5. When added together like this, it is called the **relative formula mass**. It follows that a mole of sodium chloride is 58.5 g. However, when sodium chloride is dissolved in water, it splits or ionises into its separate elements, producing a mole of sodium and a mole of chloride.

Not all relative mass formulae are straightforward additions of the relative atomic mass of the atoms because some of the molecules include water as part of their structure. For our purposes, we can ignore this water, since most of the molecules that we are concerned with are already dissolved in water.

TIME TO TRY

Using the relative atomic masses listed above, calculate the relative formula mass of the following compounds.

(a) Carbon dioxide, CO_2

    relative atomic mass of 1 atom of carbon   = _____

    relative atomic mass of 2 atoms of oxygen   = _____

    relative formula mass of 1 molecule of carbon dioxide   – _____

(b) Glucose, $C_6H_{12}O_6$

    relative atomic mass of 6 atoms of carbon   = _____

    relative atomic mass of 12 atoms of hydrogen   = _____

    relative atomic mass of 6 atoms of oxygen   = _____

    relative formula mass of 1 molecule of glucose   = _____

(c) What is the weight, in grams, of 1 mole of carbon dioxide? = _____

(d) What is the weight, in grams, of 1 mole of glucose?   = _____

Answers: (a) 44 (b) 180 (c) 44 g (d) 180 g.

If you need more practice, there are further examples at the end of the chapter.

APPLYING THE THEORY

Sodium chloride is commonly given intravenously for fluid replacement, but has to be given in amounts much smaller than a mole.

The amounts in body fluids are so small that they have to be measured in millimoles rather than moles. *There will be more about fluid replacement in Chapters 7 and 8.*

> **LOOK OUT**
>
> Intravenous fluids contain varying concentrations of the electrolytes so you must check that the fluid selected has the same strength as prescribed.

Dividing the mole

In previous chapters, you did calculations involving multiplication and division by 1000 and used the prefixes to describe divisions of the SI base units.

In the case of moles, 1 mole is divided into 1000 millimoles and 1 millimole is divided into 1000 nanomoles. See Appendix B for the table of prefixes used for SI units.

We have already established that a mole is the relative atomic mass or the relative formula mass of a substance in grams. It follows that a millimole is the relative atomic mass or the relative formula mass in milligrams.

APPLYING THE THEORY

Electrolytes in blood and intravenous fluids are measured in millimoles per litre (mmol/L). You need to recognise the normal range of the common blood values so that you can alert the right people if you are the first to see an abnormal result. A list of physiological values is given in Appendix D.

Changing millimoles to milligrams per litre

One of the common tests that are performed in the ward is the measurement of **blood glucose** levels in patients suffering from diabetes. The aim is to maintain the range between 4 and 7 mmol/L as far as possible. How do these figures relate to the mass of glucose in grams?

You have worked out that a **mole** of glucose weighs 180 g, so 1 millimole would be 180 mg and therefore:

$$4 \text{ mmol/L is equivalent to } 4 \times 180 = 720 \text{ mg/L}$$

$$7 \text{ mmol/L is equivalent to } 7 \times 180 = 1260 \text{ mg/L}$$

> **LOOK OUT**
>
> When you are reading texts or websites originating from the United States, you may see blood glucose expressed in milligrams per decilitre. A decilitre is 1/10th of a litre, i.e. 100 mL.
>
> Many of the values that we put in millimoles per litre, Americans give as **milliequivalents** per litre (mEq/L). Make sure that you are working with SI units.

KEY POINTS

● A mole is the molecular weight of a substance in grams.

● There are 1000 millimoles in 1 mole and 1000 nanomoles in 1 millimole.

● Concentrations of electrolytes and blood glucose are measured in millimoles per litre.

RUNNING WORDS

anticoagulant	formula	mole
atoms	haematuria	prophylaxis
biphasic	heparin	recombinant DNA
blood glucose	insulin	relative atomic mass
contusion	insulin syringe	relative formula mass
electrolytes	low-molecular-weight	synthetic
element	heparin	unfractionated
epistaxis	milliequivalent	units

Answers to the following questions can be found at the end of the book.

What did you learn?

How much insulin is in the following syringes if it is drawn up to the level of the arrow?

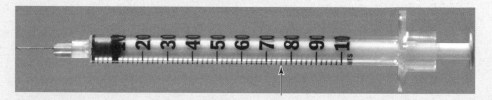

(a)

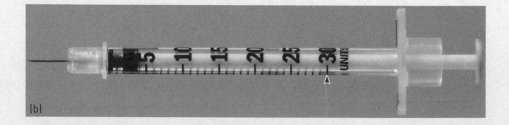

(b)

Calculate the following doses of heparin for subcutaneous injection, giving the smallest volume.

(a) 2000 units _____   (b) 9000 units _____

(c) 3000 units _____   (d) 15 000 units _____

(e) 6000 units _____   (f) 5000 units _____

More 'Time to Try' examples

Page 101
Calculate the following doses of heparin for subcutaneous injection, giving the smallest volume.

(a) 1500 units _____   (b) 3000 units _____

(c) 3500 units _____   (d) 8000 units _____

(e) 12 000 units _____   (f) 4000 units _____

Page 104
Each element has its own particular relative atomic mass (weight). Here are a few examples:

calcium	(Ca)	40
carbon	(C)	12
oxygen	(O)	16
potassium	(K)	39
sodium	(Na)	23
chlorine	(Cl)	35.5

Use the relative atomic masses above to calculate the following relative formula mass of the following compounds.

(a) Potassium chloride, KCl

relative atomic mass of 1 atom of potassium = _____

relative atomic mass of 1 atom of chlorine = _____

relative formula mass of 1 molecule of potassium chloride = _____

(b) Calcium carbonate, $CaCO_3$

relative atomic mass of 1 atom of calcium = _____

relative atomic mass of 1 atom of carbon = _____

relative atomic mass of 3 atoms of oxygen = _____

relative formula mass of 1 molecule of calcium carbonate = _____

(c) What is the weight, in grams, of 1 mole of potassium chloride? _____

(d) What is the weight, in grams, of 1 mole of calcium carbonate? _____

Web resources

http://www.moleday.org/
A totally over the top website but fun!

http://news.bbc.co.uk/1/hi/health/7379546.stm
A cautionary tale about the accuracy of equipment.

http://www.bbc.co.uk/scotland/education/bitesize/higher/chemistry/calculations_1/mole_rev.shtm
Moles and molar solutions.

http://www.nursingtimes.net/This_weeks_issue/2008/01/how_do_we_reduce_drug_errors.html
An insight into drug errors and how to prevent them.

http://www.diabeteshealth.com/read/2002/11/01/3039.html
Insulin error in misreading the prescription.

www.bddiabetes.com/us/hcp/main.aspx
Go to the section on prescribing insulin syringes and look at the rationale for choosing a particular syringe.

Chapter 6

Per cent, percentage and ratios

Hundreds and thousands and much more

Some drug strengths are expressed as a percentage and solutions used for the treatment of some skin conditions are diluted from a concentrated solution.

A number of returns that have to be made about bed occupancy, patient admissions and types of conditions that caused admission are required as percentages. It is also handy in everyday life to be able to understand per cent when seeking a bargain.

When you have completed this chapter, you should be able to:

- Change vulgar and decimal fractions to per cent.

- Calculate percentages.

- Use a calculator to calculate per cent.

- Calculate the amount of drug in a percentage solution.

- Prepare a solution to a given ratio or concentration.

6.1 PER CENT

YOUR STARTING POINT FOR PER CENT

Express the following as percentages.

(a) 1/2 = _____   (b) 1/20 = _____

(c) 1/5 = _____   (d) 3/4 = _____

Write the following as vulgar fractions in their simplest form.

(e) 35% = _____   (f) 56% = _____   (g) 72% = _____

What are the following?

(h) 10% of 250 = _____   (i) 20% of 440 = _____   (j) 30% of 210 = _____

Convert these decimal fractions to percentages.

(k) 0.3 = _____   (l) 0.15 = _____   (m) 0.37 = _____

Change these percentages to decimal fractions.

(n) 34% = _____   (o) 29% = _____   (p) 7% = _____

What percentage is the first number of the second?

(q) 500 out of 2000 = _____   (r) 26 out of 208 = _____

(s) 200 out of 8000 = _____

Answers: (a) 50% (b) 5% (c) 20% (d) 75% (e) 7/20 (f) 14/25 (g) 18/25 (h) 25 (i) 88 (j) 63 (k) 30% (l) 15% (m) 37% (n) 0.34 (o) 0.29 (p) 0.07 (q) 25% (r) 12.5% (s) 2.5%.

If you had these all correct, skip through to Section 6.2.

What is per cent?

Per cent means 'parts per hundred'. You are already familiar with your examination marks being given as a per cent – marks out of 100. Since per cent is out of 100, this means that it is a fraction of 100.

There are several ways of indicating per cent, e.g. 1 per cent can be written as a vulgar fraction 1/100, as a decimal fraction 0.01 or as the familiar 1%. It follows that 45% means 45 parts out of 100 or 45/100.

You may sometimes need to calculate a **percentage** from two numbers. For example, what percentage of 2500 is 150?

Take 2500 as the 100%, so to calculate the percentage represented by 150 say the sum out aloud '150 out of 2500', and write it down as if it were one of your exam marks:

$$\frac{150}{2500}$$

Now all you need to do is to multiply it by 100 to convert it to a percentage. So

$$\frac{150}{2500} \times 100 = 6\%$$

Per cent is a tidy way to present results and is easier to compare **data**.

EXAMPLE

Patients in each of three wards were asked if they preferred to have a hot drink just before lights out or earlier in the evening. Ward A of 28 patients had 3 who preferred the early option, ward B of 21 patients had 7 and ward C of 36 patients had 9.

It is easier to compare data when presented as a percentage. If we need to convert the results to per cent, the first thing we have to do is to make a fraction of the data given: in ward A, 3 out of 28 patients, which is 3/28, in ward B, 7/21 and in ward C, 9/36.

To convert these vulgar fractions to percentages you just need to multiply the fraction by 100:

ward A: $\dfrac{3}{28} \times 100 = 10.7\%$ ward B: $\dfrac{7}{21} \times 100 = 33.3\%$ ward C: $\dfrac{9}{36} \times 100 = 25\%$

 If you have difficulty in following the calculation, go back to the section on multiplication of fractions in Chapter 2.

You can compare any numbers by putting them into percentage form. As you saw in the example above, what you need to do is to put the smaller number over the larger one as a vulgar fraction and then multiply the fraction by 100 to give you the percentage.

EXAMPLE

What is 250 as a percentage of 2000?

First make an improper fraction, 250/2000, then multiply it by 100 to make a percentage:

$$\frac{250}{2000} \times 100 = 12.5\%$$

Reversing the process ...

 To change a percentage to a vulgar fraction, first put the percentage over 100 and then reduce the fraction to its lowest terms. *Look at Chapter 2 if you need to refresh your skills at reducing fractions.*

EXAMPLES

(a) What is 50% as a fraction?

$$\frac{50}{100} \text{ both numbers can be divided by 10} = \frac{5}{10}$$

$$\frac{5}{10} \text{ both numbers can be divided by 5} = \frac{1}{2}$$

(b) What is 40% as a fraction?

$$\frac{40}{100} = \frac{4}{10} = \frac{2}{5}$$

TIME TO TRY

Change the following vulgar fractions to percentages correct to one decimal place where the answer is not a whole number.

(a) 2/20 = _____ %   (b) 1/5 = _____ %   (c) 5/15 = _____ %

(d) 3/4 = _____ %   (e) 1/2 = _____ %   (f) 1/3 = _____ %

(g) 1/40 = _____ %   (h) 6/20 = _____ %

Answers: (a) 10% (b) 20% (c) 33.3% (d) 75% (e) 50% (f) 33.3% (g) 2.5% (h) 30%.

Change the following percentages to vulgar fractions in their lowest terms.

(a) 25% = _____   (b) 75% = _____   (c) 35% = _____

(d) 60% = _____   (e) 56% = _____   (f) 44% = _____

(g) 15% = _____   (h) $33\frac{1}{3}$% = _____

Answers: (a) 1/4 (b) 3/4 (c) 7/20 (d) 3/5 (e) 14/25 (f) 11/25 (g) 3/20 (h) 1/3.

If you need more practice, there are further examples at the end of the chapter.

How do you find a percentage of a number?

At sale time, bargains are often displayed as saving you a percentage of the original price, say 20% off. The first thing that you need to ask is 'Off what?' You can then work out the actual amount that you are saving.

EXAMPLE

A pair of Jimmy Choo shoes is advertised as '20% off previous price'. The previous price was £360. You can now work out how much you will save and how much you will have to pay.

If you say the question out loud, 'What is 20 per cent of £360?', you will be able to set out the calculation easily, especially if you have remembered that 'of' means multiply.

Write 20% as a vulgar fraction and then multiply by the number that represents 100%:

$$\frac{20}{100} \times £360 = £72$$

You have now found that you can save £72 off the original price, so you have to pay

$$£360 - £72 = £288 \quad \text{(not bad for a pair of Jimmy Choos)}$$

APPLYING THE THEORY

You are offered 15% discount if you buy 12 electronic thermometers costing £18.80 each. You receive a quote from another manufacturer offering you 20% discount on the same quantity but these cost £19.20. Which is the better deal?

Find the amount that represents 15% of £18.80:

$$\frac{15}{100} \times £18.80 = £2.82$$

This means that each thermometer will cost

$$£18.80 - £2.82 = £15.98$$

Now work out the saving on the other quote of 20% of £19.20:

$$\frac{20}{100} \times £19.20 = £3.84$$

The cost of each thermometer will be

$$£19.20 - £3.84 = £15.36$$

Now you have worked out the percentages, you will see that the second quote is better by 62 pence per thermometer.

APPLYING THE THEORY

During your course, you will be asked to read papers which you have to use in writing assignments. Not all papers are clear at first reading and it is useful if you can do some calculations so that the information is more meaningful.

Many reports present information as a percentage: for example, in 2003, cardiovascular disease (CVD) caused 39% of deaths in the UK. The percentage does not give you any idea of how many people that represents.

To make more sense of these **statistics**, you need to know that the total number of deaths for that year was 612000. To find the number of people who died from CVD, you now know that 612000 was 100% of all deaths, so you can find out what number is represented by 39%:

$$\frac{39}{100} \times 612000 = 238680 \text{ deaths from CVD}$$

You will be learning more about making sense of statistics in Chapter 10.

TIME TO TRY

Find the number that is represented by the following percentages, correct to one decimal place.

(a) 25% of 40 = _____   (b) 35% of 450 = _____

(c) 43% of 1240 = _____   (d) 62% of 372 = _____

(e) 53% of 625 = _____   (f) 12% of 250 = _____

Find the saving if the following discounts are offered.

(g) 20% off £ 5.50 = _____

(h) 15% off £27.00 = _____

(i) 17.5% off £14.00 = _____

(j) 12.5% off £16 = _____

(k) 45% off £72.00 = _____

(l) 22% off £53.00 = _____

Answers: (a) 10 (b) 157.5 (c) 533.2 (d) 230.6 (e) 331.3 (f) 30 (g) £1.10 (h) £4.05 (i) £2.45
(j) £2.00 (k) £32.40 (l) £11.66.

If you need more practice, there are further examples at the end of the chapter.

> **KEY POINTS**
>
> - To convert a vulgar fraction to a percentage, multiply the fraction by 100.
> - To convert a percentage to a vulgar fraction, put the percentage over 100 and reduce to its simplest form.
> - To find out the number represented by a percentage, write the percentage as a vulgar fraction out of 100 and multiply the fraction by the number that represents 100%.
> - To find the percentage that one number is of another number, put the smaller number over the larger one and multiply by 100.

Decimal fractions and percentages

Converting a **decimal fraction** to a percentage is straightforward – you simply multiply the decimal fraction by 100. For example, 0.7 as a percentage is

$$0.7 \times 100 = 70\%$$

To change a percentage to a decimal fraction, just divide the percentage by 100. For example, 43% as a decimal fraction is

$$43 \div 100 = 0.43$$

If you can't remember how to multiply and divide by 100, see Chapter 2.

TIME TO TRY

Change the following decimal fractions to percentages.

(a) 0.25 = _____ %   (b) 0.4 = _____ %   (c) 0.04 = _____ %   (d) 0.38 = _____ %

Change the following percentages to decimal fractions.

(e) 75% = _____   (f) 33% = _____   (g) 5% = _____   (h) 61% = _____

Answers: (a) 25% (b) 40% (c) 4% (d) 38% (e) 0.75 (f) 0.33 (g) 0.05 (h) 0.61.

If you need more practice, there are further examples at the end of the chapter.

6.2 PERCENTAGE CONCENTRATION

YOUR STARTING POINT FOR PERCENTAGE CONCENTRATION

Calculate the weight, in grams, of the substance dissolved in the following volumes of solution.

(a) 500 mL of a 5% w/v solution of glucose = _____

(b) 1 L of 0.9% w/v sodium chloride = _____

(c) 10 mL of 15% w/v potassium chloride = _____

(d) 100 mL of 8.4% w/v sodium bicarbonate = _____

How many millilitres of the following drugs are needed to give the required dose?

(e) Dose required is 100 mg of a 2% w/v solution = _____

(f) Dose required is 50 mg of a 0.5% w/v solution = _____

(g) Dose required is 250 mg of a 20% w/v solution = _____

(h) Dose required is 200 mg of a 4% w/v solution = _____

What weight of active ingredient is in the following skin preparations?

(i) 100 g of 3% w/w hydrocortisone cream = _____

(j) 50 g of 2% w/w dithranol ointment = _____

(k) What volume of 20% concentrated solution do you need to make 200 mL of a 10% solution? _____

(l) What volume of 10% concentrated solution do you need to make 300 mL of a 2% solution? _____

Answers: (a) 25 g (b) 9 g (c) 1.5 g (d) 8.4 g (e) 5 mL (f) 10 mL (g) 1.25 mL (h) 5 mL (i) 3 g (j) 1 g (k) 100 mL (l) 60 mL

If you had all of these correct, move on to Section 6.3. If you are unsure of how to do these calculations, then work through the following section.

Percentage concentrations

There are different ways of expressing the concentration of drugs, depending on the type of medication and the route through which it is given. You have already carried out calculations where the drug is measured in grams or milligrams per millilitre and those special drugs measured in units.

We are now going to look at drug concentrations that are expressed as percentages.

Percentage concentrations can take three forms: **weight in volume (w/v)**, **weight in weight (w/w)** or **volume in volume (v/v)**.

An important point to remember is that when we compare weight and volume 1 litre of water weighs 1 kilogram. (You might get into an argument with a scientist, but for our purposes this is fine.) If 1 litre of water weighs 1 kilogram, 1000 milli-litres (1 L) weighs 1000 grams (1 kg) and so 1 mL weighs 1 g.

Percentage concentration is used when a solid is dissolved in water (w/v) and refers to the number of grams dissolved in 100 mL (which weighs 100 g).

The percentage solution is written as % w/v; for example, sodium chloride solution for intravenous infusion is in a concentration of 0.9% w/v. This means that 0.9 g is dissolved in every 100 mL of water.

Normally, bags of intravenous fluid contain 500 mL or 1 L of solution. If you need to work out how much sodium chloride is contained in a 1 L bag then you can use the method that we used earlier to work out percentages.

Write out the percentage as a vulgar fraction

$$\frac{0.9 \text{ g}}{100}$$

then multiply it by the volume of fluid, in millilitres, to be given:

$$\frac{0.9 \text{ g}}{100 \text{ mL}} \times 1000 \text{ mL} = \frac{900 \text{ g}}{100} = 9 \text{ g}$$

From this calculation, you can see that a litre of 0.9% sodium chloride contains 9 g of sodium chloride.

Skin conditions are a common problem encountered in clinical practice, from simple rashes to chronic problems such as eczema. Topical creams and ointments are normally prescribed and the active ingredient is usually expressed as % w/w. Here it means the number of grams of the active ingredient that are mixed in 100 g of the base cream or ointment.

Some creams are very potent and there is a weekly limit to the total amount used. Again the same method can be used to calculate the weight of active ingre-dient used.

If a cream has a concentration of 2.5% w/w and a patient uses 200 g every week, then the total amount of drug used is the concentration as a vulgar fraction

$$\frac{2.5 \text{ g}}{100 \text{ g}}$$

multiplied by the total weight of the cream used

$$\frac{2.5 \text{ g}}{100 \text{ g}} \times 200 \text{ g} = 5 \text{ g}$$

Over the week the patient has received 5 g of the active ingredient.

% v/v is much less frequently found in practice. It is the percentage of a liquid, in millilitres, mixed into 100 millilitres of another liquid. You may use this type of cal-culation when you dilute a concentrated liquid (often called a stock solution) with water to make a weaker solution.

Chlorhexadine 5% is an antiseptic solution in concentrated form. It needs to be diluted to activate its antiseptic properties and to prevent toxic effects. The normal concentration for use as a skin antiseptic is 0.05% v/v so you need to calculate how much of the concentrate needs to be diluted.

If there is 5 g of chlorhexadine in 100 mL and what you need is 200 mL of 0.05 g in 100 mL, divide the dilute strength by the concentrated strength and multiply by the total volume of the diluted solution that you need:

$$\frac{0.05 \text{ g}}{5 \text{ g}} \times 200 \text{ mL} = 2 \text{ mL}$$

You will need to measure 2 mL of the stock solution and add 198 mL of water to obtain 200 mL of a 0.05% concentration.

APPLYING THE THEORY

When a patient is going to undergo a potentially painful procedure such as removal of a cyst, the area will be made numb with a local anaesthetic. **Lidocaine** is one of the common drugs used for this purpose. You may have had some if you have had a root filling at the dentist.

There is a limit to the amount of drug that can be given without the risk of toxic effects. Lidocaine is produced in concentrations of 0.5%, 1% and 2%. The dose is based on the patient's weight and a maximum recommended dose of 200 mg, so it is important that a check is kept on the volume and strength of the drug so that the patient does not have an overdose, especially if a further dose has to be given to complete the procedure.

If 10 mL of a 1% solution is given, how many milligrams will the patient receive?

Now 1% means that there is 1 g of the drug in 100 mL, so make these figures into a vulgar fraction and change grams to milligrams:

$$\frac{1 \text{ g}}{100 \text{ mL}} = \frac{1000 \text{ mg}}{100 \text{ mL}} = 10 \text{ mg}/1 \text{ mL}$$

So in 10 mL there is 10×10 mg/mL = 100 mg which is half the recommended dose.

> **LOOK OUT**
> Make sure that you check the patient's weight so that the correct dose can be given.

Calculating a dose from a percentage solution

Patients suffering from diabetes may sometimes take their insulin or glucose-lowering tablets but miss a meal or do not eat enough carbohydrate to meet their needs. The result is that their blood glucose drops too low and they urgently need some glucose to prevent their going into a coma.

Glucose solution can be given orally or a special preparation can be given into a vein for a very rapid action. A record of how many grams of glucose given must be made and so it is important to be able to calculate the amount in each dose.

EXAMPLE

If 200 mL of a 20% solution is given to a patient, how much glucose has the patient received?

You already know that a 20% solution contains 20 g in 100 ml of liquid. To calculate the amount of glucose in 200 mL, first change the percentage to a vulgar fraction and multiply by the volume prescribed:

$$\frac{20 \text{ g}}{100 \text{ mL}} \times 200 \text{ mL} = 40 \text{ g}$$

It is also possible that the patient is prescribed the dose in grams or milligrams.

For example, 50 g of glucose is prescribed to be given as an intravenous injection. What volume of a 20% solution will you need for this dose?

Make the percentage into a vulgar fraction:

$$\frac{20 \text{ g}}{100 \text{ mL}}$$

which means that every 100 mL contains 20 g of glucose.

If you carry out the division you will find that 1 mL contains 0.2 g, so to find the number of millilitres needed to give a 50 g dose you need to find how many 'lots' of 0.2 g there are in 50 g. To do that you divide 50 g by 0.2 g = 250 mL.

You can calculate it all as one sum:

$$50 \text{ g} \div \frac{20 \text{ g}}{100 \text{ mL}} = 50 \text{ g} \times \frac{100 \text{ mL}}{20 \text{ g}} = \frac{5000 \text{ mL}}{20} = 250 \text{ mL}$$

 If you have forgotten how to divide by fractions, look at Chapter 2.

> ### KEY POINTS
>
> **Percentage concentrations can be expressed in different forms:**
>
> - Weight in weight, w/w
> - Weight in volume, w/v
> - Volume in volume, v/v.

TIME TO TRY

Calculate the weight, in grams, of the substance dissolved in the following volumes of solution.

(a) 1 L of a 5% w/v solution of glucose = _____

(b) 500 mL of 0.9% w/v sodium chloride = _____

(c) 10 mL of 10% w/v potassium chloride = __ _____

(d) 500 mL of 8.4% w/v sodium bicarbonate = _____

How many millilitres of the following drugs are needed to give the required dose?

(e) Dose required is 75 mg of a 5% w/v solution = _____

(f) Dose required is 250 mg of a 1% w/v solution = _____

(g) Dose required is 500 mg of a 10% w/v solution = _____

(h) Dose required is 150 mg of a 4% w/v solution = _____

What weight of active ingredient is in the following skin preparations?

(i) 100 g of 2% w/w hydrocortisone cream = _____

(j) 50 g of 1% w/w dithranol ointment = _____

(k) What volume of 40% concentrated solution do you need to make 200 mL of a 20% solution? _____

(l) What volume of 10% concentrated solution do you need to make 300 mL of a 1% solution? _____

Answers: (a) 50 g (b) 4.5 g (c) 1 g (d) 4.2 g (e) 1.5 mL (f) 25 mL (g) 5 mL (h) 3.75 mL (i) 2 g (j) 0.5 g (k) 100 mL (l) 30 mL.

If you need more practice, there are further examples at the end of the chapter.

How to use your calculator to work out percentages

There are numerous models of calculator ranging from simple ones (**Figure 6.1**) to **scientific calculators** that are programmable. The simplest types are adequate for the purposes of drug calculations but if you are going to have to work out statistics

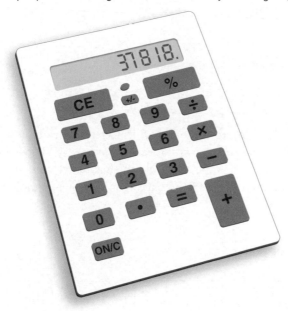

Figure 6.1 Basic calculator with % key

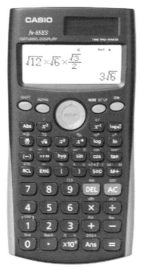

Figure 6.2 Non-programmable scientific calculator

Source: Casio

or calculations involving exponents, then a basic scientific calculator may be more useful (**Figure 6.2**).

The following instructions will suit most calculators but you need to make sure that you understand how yours works and that, if you have a scientific calculator, are operating it in the correct mode.

The simple calculator (Figure 6.1) has a % key, so it is a quick way of doing the sum. It is important that you put in the information in the correct order, otherwise the answer may be wrong.

EXAMPLE

What is 15% of 75? Enter the numbers like this:

$$\boxed{1}\ \boxed{5}\ \boxed{\times}\ \boxed{7}\ \boxed{5}\ \boxed{\%}$$

There is usually no need to press the = key; in fact this may lead to an incorrect answer, but with some older calculators this may be necessary – know your calculator.

If there is no % button, as is the case with the scientific calculator (Figure 6.2), then enter the whole sum making 15% into a vulgar fraction and multiplying it by 75:

$$\frac{15}{100} \times 75$$

Enter the numbers like this:

$$\boxed{1}\ \boxed{5}\ \boxed{\times}\ \boxed{7}\ \boxed{5}\ \boxed{\div}\ \boxed{1}\ \boxed{0}\ \boxed{0}\ \boxed{=}$$

The answer is the same, 11.25, whichever method you use.

6.3 RATIOS

YOUR STARTING POINT FOR RATIOS

How much concentrate do you need to make the following dilutions?

(a) 200 mL of a 1 in 4 solution = _____ (b) 300 mL of a 1:5 solution = _____

What volume of adrenaline 1 in 1000 do you need to give the following doses?

(c) 250 micrograms = _____ (d) 100 micrograms = _____

Which of the following ratios is the odd one out?

(e) 25:100, 4:16, 3:9, 180:720 _____ (f) 9:27, 3:9, 8:28, 25:75 _____

Answers: (a) 50 mL (b) 50 mL (c) 0.25 mL (d) 0.1 mL (e) 3:9 (f) 8:28.

As you have seen, there are various ways to write the concentration of drugs and medicinal products. Just to keep everyone on their toes, there is another method of stating the strength of a solution, and that is as a **ratio**:

ratios are written in the form of **1 in** 4, **1:**4 or **1 to** 4

A 1 in 4 solution means that 1 part out of every 4 is the concentrated solution and is mixed with 3 parts of the diluent.

The ratios 1:4 and 1 to 4 mean the same thing: 1 to 4 means that every 1 part of concentrate is mixed with 4 parts of the diluent, making a total of 5 parts (since there are five portions in total, it could also be written as a 1 in 5 solution).

It is important to know which is which, as they will give different results. You will notice the difference if you experiment with orange squash. Try a dilution of 1 measure of squash with 3 measures of water, a 1 in 4 solution or 1 measure of squash with 4 measures of water, a 1 to 4 (1:4) or even a 1 in 5 solution!

You will also see ratios used in reports, such as the number of people who have a mobile phone or the number of teachers to students in a school.

If you count the number of male and female students in your cohort, you may find that the ratio is something like 24 to 60. If the cohort before yours has a ratio of 32:80 it is difficult to compare it directly. When you had vulgar fractions, they could be simplified so that they were easier to handle; ratios can also be simplified.

The same rules apply here as with the simplification of vulgar fractions: the same process must be applied to both numbers. Both numbers of the ratio 24:60 can be divided by 12 to leave the ratio 2:5. The second ratio 32:80 can be divided by 16 to give 2:5, so both cohorts have the same ratio of males to females.

APPLYING THE THEORY

Adrenaline (epinephrine) is given in emergencies such as an allergic reaction or circulatory failure. The concentration of the drug is written as a ratio. It comes in strengths of 1 in 1000 or 1 in 10000. In a 1 in 1000 adrenaline ampoule there is

1 part adrenaline in 999 parts and in a 1 in 10 000 ampoule there is 1 part adrenaline in 9999 parts of solution.

To work out how many milligrams of adrenaline are present:

1 in 1000 solution adrenaline (remember that 1 mL of water weighs 1 g)

1 g adrenaline is in 1000 mL of solution = 1000 mg adrenaline per 1000 mL and so 1 mg per mL

How many micrograms of adrenaline are there in a 1 in 10 000 solution? = _____

1 g adrenaline in 10 000 mL solution

1000 mg per 10 000 mL

0.1 mg per 1 mL which is 100 micrograms per mL

  If you have forgotten how to change one SI unit to another, look at Chapter 3.

LOOK OUT

Ampoules of 1 in 1000 and 1 in 10 000 look very similar. The weaker solution (1 in 10 000) is generally for intravenous use. If the 1 in 1000 solution is used, the patient can suffer a severe rise in blood pressure and heart rate.

The labelling of adrenaline is under review, since working out the dose in milligrams or micrograms from a ratio solution takes time and is prone to error (University of Cambridge, 2008).

APPLYING THE THEORY

Dermatologists may prescribe potassium permanganate to be applied as wet soaks or baths for patients with weeping eczema. This product needs to be very dilute, since it can cause irritation to mucous membranes.

The tablets are 400 mg each and the concentration required is 1 in 10 000 solution. A 1 in 10 000 solution, as we saw above, is 0.1 mg per mL.

Potassium permanganate tablets are 400 mg each. If there is 0.1 mg in 1 mL, in a 1 in 10 000 solution, to find the volume needed for 400 mg:

$$\frac{400 \text{ mg}}{0.1 \text{ mg}} \times 1 \text{ mL} = 4000 \text{ mL} = 4 \text{ L}$$

LOOK OUT

Potassium permanganate stains skin and clothing brown. It should not be used if there are open wounds and soaking should be for a maximum of 10 minutes to prevent absorption through mucous membranes.

KEY POINTS

Ratios:

- Ratios show the relationships between two or more items.
- 1 in 10 means 1 part in a total of 10 parts.
- 1:10 and 1 to 10 mean that 1 portion is added to 10 portions making a total of 11 parts.
- Solutions 1 in 1000 mean that there is 1 g in 1000 mL or 1000 mg in 1000 mL, which is equivalent to 1 mg/mL.

TIME TO TRY

How much concentrate do you need to make the following dilutions?

(a) 500 mL of a 1 in 4 solution = _____   (b) 600 mL of a 1:5 solution = _____

What volume of adrenaline 1 in 1000 do you need to give the following doses?

(c) 500 micrograms = _____   (d) 120 micrograms = _____

Which of the following ratios is the odd one out?

(e) 25:100, 4:16, 3:9, 180:720 = _____   (f) 9:27, 3:9, 8:28, 25:75 = _____

Answers: (a) 125 mL (b) 100 mL (c) 0.5 mL (d) 0.12 mL (e) 3:9 (f) 8:28.

If you need more practice, there are further examples at the end of the chapter.

RUNNING WORDS

1 in ...	decimal fractions	statistics
1 to ...	lidocaine	volume/volume, v/v
1: ...	per cent	weight/volume, w/v
adrenaline (epinephrine)	percentage	weight/weight, w/w
chlorhexadine	ratio	
data	scientific calculator	

Answers to the following questions can be found at the end of the book.

What did you learn?

Change the following to a percentage.

(a) 1/5 = _____%   (b) 0.04 = _____

Change the following to decimal fractions.

(c) 43% = _____   (d) 1/20 = _____

Calculate the following percentages.

(e) 30% of 180 = _____   (f) 17.5% of £3.00 = _____

(g) 87% of 2 litres = _____   (h) 5% of 500 g = _____

How much water do you need to make the following dilutions?

(i) 1 in 10 000 solution of potassium permanganate using 400 mg tablets =

_____

(j) 500 mL of a 1 in 100 solution = _____

(k) 1.5 L of a 1 to 4 solution = _____

What volume of 1 in 10 000 solution of adrenaline contains the following doses?

(l) 100 micrograms = _____   (m) 250 micrograms = _____

How many grams of solute are dissolved in the following solutions?

(n) 1 L of 10% glucose = _____

(o) 250 mL of 0.9% sodium chloride = _____

More 'Time to Try' examples

Page 112

Change the following vulgar fractions to percentages correct to one decimal place where the answer is not a whole number.

(a) 1/10 = _____%   (b) 3/5 = _____%   (c) 4/30 = _____%

(d) 5/8 = _____%   (e) 1/4 = _____%   (f) 2/3 = _____%

(g) 1/50 = _____%   (h) 1/20 = _____%

Change the following percentages to vulgar fractions in their lowest terms.

(i) 22% = _____   (j) 85% = _____   (k) 40% = _____

(l) 30% = _____   (m) 46% = _____   (n) 55% = _____

(o) 12% = _____   (p) 64% = _____

Page 113–114

Find the number that is represented by the following percentages, correct to one decimal place where the answer is not a whole number.

(a) 55% of 50 = _____   (b) 30% of 250 = _____

(c) 34% of 1130 = _____   (d) 46% of 366 = _____

(e) 67% of 960 = _____   (f) 24% of 550 = _____

Find the saving if the following discounts are offered.

(g) 10% off £17.50 = _____   (h) 25% off £37.00 = _____

(i) 17.5% off £14.00 = _____   (j) 12.5 % off £16 = _____

(k) 45% off £72.00 = _____   (l) 22% off £53.00 = _____

Page 114

Change the following percentages to decimal fractions.

(a) 63% = _____   (b) 37% = _____

(c) 2% = _____   (d) 59% = _____

Change the following decimal fractions to percentages.

(e) 0.35 = _____%   (f) 0.07 = _____%

(g) 0.19 = _____%   (h) 0.62 = _____%

Page 118-119

Calculate the weight, in grams, of the substance dissolved in the following volumes of solution.

(a) 500 mL of a 10% w/v solution of glucose = _____

(b) 1000 mL of 0.9% w/v sodium chloride = _____

(c) 10 mL of 5% w/v potassium chloride = _____

(d) 250 mL of 8.4% w/v sodium bicarbonate = _____

How many millilitres of the following drugs are needed to give the required dose?

(e) Dose required is 125 mg of a 5% w/v solution = _____

(f) Dose required is 300 mg of a 1% w/v solution = _____

(g) Dose required is 500 mg of a 10% w/v solution = _____

(h) Dose required is 150 mg of a 5% w/v solution = _____

What weight of active ingredient is in the following skin preparations?

(i) 150 g of 2% w/w hydrocortisone cream = _____

(j) 50 g of 2% w/w dithranol ointment = _____

(k) What volume of 0.1% concentrated solution do you need to make 200 mL of a 0.01% solution? _____

(l) What volume of 10% concentrated solution do you need to make 150 mL of a 1% solution? _____

Page 123

How much concentrate do you need to make the following dilutions?

(a) 300 mL of a 1 in 5 solution = _____

(b) 400 mL of a 1:3 solution = _____

What volume of adrenaline 1 in 1000 do you need to give the following doses?

(c) 250 micrograms = _____

(d) 50 micrograms = _____

Which of the following ratios is the odd one out?

(e) 24:96, 7:28, 9:18, 16:64 = _____

(f) 6:18, 8:24, 4:14, 20:60 = _____

Web resources

http://www.bbc.co.uk/schools/ks3bitesize/maths/number/index.shtml
The section on ratios gives several examples, including map scales which could be useful for hill walking.

http://edhelper.com/percents.htm
Practice examples of converting per cent to decimal fractions, decimal fractions to per cent and ratios as percentages.

http://learntech.uwe.ac.uk/numeracy/
Practice for a wide variety of numeracy skills for drug calculations, including animations of ratios.

Reference

University of Cambridge (2008) Doctors may be giving wrong dosage of adrenaline in an emergency because of labelling. *ScienceDaily*. Retrieved 21 June 2008, from http://www.sciencedaily.com/releases/2008/01/080101093858.htm.

Chapter 7

Intravenous fluid and drug administration

Drips, drops and devices

Intravenous fluids are prescribed and so need to be treated as any
other prescription medicine. It is therefore necessary to be able
to calculate accurately the rate at which the fluid should be given.
IV fluids, as they are often known, are a common method of
rehydrating patients. This chapter will teach you how to do these
calculations.

When you have completed this chapter, you should be able to:

- Calculate the infusion rate for a manually regulated infusion.
- Calculate the infusion rate using infusion pumps.
- Calculate the dose of drug to be given via a syringe driver.
- Calculate the rate of flow for a blood transfusion.
- Identify the potential problems associated with these methods of
  administration.

Approximately 60% of an adult's body weight is composed of water containing dissolved salts. A lean person has a higher proportion of water in their body than an obese individual.

Some of this fluid is circulating as blood, another portion is bathing the cells of the tissues and organs, but by far the largest volume is inside the cells.

Fluid is lost from the body on a daily basis through urine, sweat and respiration. Normally fluid output is balanced by fluid intake from drinks and food but in some circumstances such as haemorrhage, diarrhoea and vomiting, or other severe fluid loss, replacement is needed via an intravenous infusion.

 There will be more about fluid balance in Chapter 8.

As people get older, their percentage of body fluid is reduced to as little as 45% by the age of 80 years. Fluid loss will have a greater impact on their general well-being so it is important to ensure that their fluid intake is maintained.

Small children have a fluid content of 70–80% and can become dehydrated very quickly.

The **intravenous (IV)** route is used whenever a patient is unable to take in sufficient fluid by mouth because the patient is too weak, unconscious or unable to tolerate anything orally. It is not the first choice because there are a number of potential problems associated with intravenous access, which will be discussed later in the chapter.

7.1 INTRAVENOUS INFUSION

A suitable cannula has to be inserted into a vein by a qualified practitioner, so that an intravenous administration set can be attached in order to give the prescribed fluids.

Before attaching the administration set or giving further fluid, the cannula site should be checked for any signs of inflammation, swelling, leakage or symptoms of pain or discomfort.

Intravenous fluids are normally presented in clear plastic bags which have a port for connection to the administration set and are wrapped in an outer bag for security (**Figure 7.1**). A standard administration set is used to give fluids manually (**Figure 7.2**).

> **LOOK OUT**
>
> Check the fluid with the prescription, the expiry date and make sure that the outer pack is undamaged and does not contain condensation. After opening the outer bag of the fluid, check that the fluid does not contain any crystals which may occur if the fluid has been badly stored. The packaging of the giving set should be checked for damage and its expiry date.

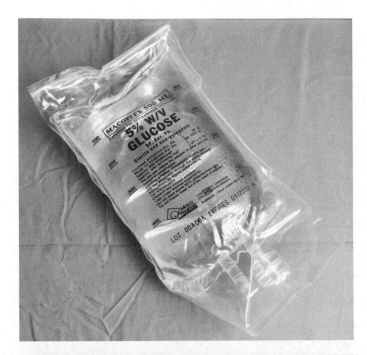

Figure 7.1
A 1 litre bag of
5% glucose in
outer wrapping
Source: Mediscan

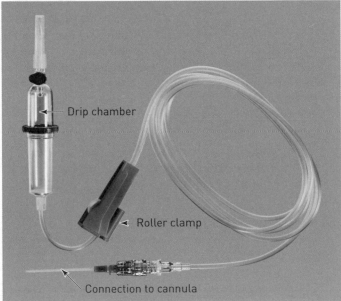

Drip chamber

Roller clamp

Connection to cannula

Figure 7.2
A standard
administration
(giving) set
Source: Wellcome Images

The type of infusion device needs to be considered, since there are a variety of pumps available, each with different characteristics. The choice will depend on the risk level of the infusions as well as the types that are available in the clinical setting. The delivery set must be matched to the infusion pump, so it is important to know your equipment and how it works.

Pumps deliver fluids in millilitres per hour (**Figure 7.3**) whereas the manual method must be calculated in **drops per minute**. You may come across some older

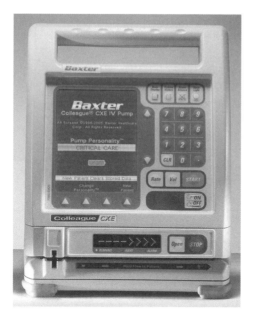

Figure 7.3 An example of a volumetric infusion pump

Source: Baxter Healthcare Ltd

machines that deliver drops per minute but they are unreliable and are no longer manufactured.

Whichever method of delivery is used, a calculation needs to be made in order to obtain the correct flow rate.

A manually regulated system consists of the bag of fluid, the administration set (also known as a giving set) and the cannula which has been inserted and secured in place (**Figure 7.4**).

Intravenous fluids must be prescribed, just as any other medication (**Table 7.1**). The type, concentration and volume of fluid are specified as well as the period of time over which it has to be given. The volume of fluid must be given at a steady pace over the time prescribed, so it is important to know how to calculate the infusion rate. (Also see the example of a drug administration sheet in Appendix F.)

The standard administration set delivers 20 drops per millilitre of fluid,

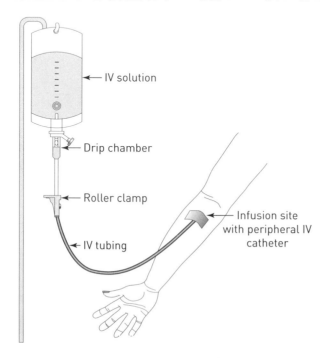

← IV solution

← Drip chamber

← Roller clamp

← IV tubing

← Infusion site with peripheral IV catheter

Figure 7.4 The setup of the basic, manually controlled, gravity-assisted infusion

Source: Olsen, J. *et al.* (2008) *Medical Dosage Calculations*, Prentice Hall

Table 7.1 Example of a prescription for intravenous fluid

Date	Intravenous fluid	Volume	Duration	Additive and dose	Prescriber's signature	Batch number	Nurse's signature	Time started	Time completed
01.01.01	0.9% sodium chloride	1 litre	6 hours	None	A.Doctor				

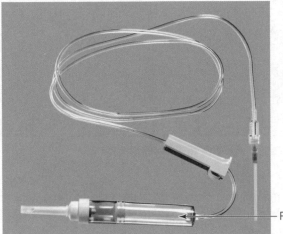

Filter in chamber

Figure 7.5 A blood administration set with filter chamber

Source: Wellcome Images

but those used for blood products are calibrated to give 15 drops per millilitre and also have a second chamber containing a filter (**Figure 7.5**).

There are special sets that are used for paediatric infusions and for the delivery of some intravenous drugs. These sets deliver 60 drops per millilitre and are known as micro-drop **burettes** (**Figure 7.6**).

If you are unsure about the number of drops per millilitre of the set you are about to use, then check the information on the packaging.

It is not within the scope of this book to show you how to set up the equipment, but to focus on the arithmetic involved in calculating the rate of infusion. It is vital for you to understand the calculation before you assist in setting up the equipment.

YOUR STARTING POINT FOR CALCULATING INFUSION RATE

Calculate the following infusion rate in drops per minute (dpm) if the fluid is to be given intravenously via a **standard administration set** that delivers 20 drops per millilitre (correct to the nearest whole drop).

(a) 500 mL of 5% glucose over 3 hours = _____

(b) 100 mL Metronidazole over 1/2 hour = _____

(c) 1 L sodium chloride 0.45% with 2.5% glucose over 4 hours = _____

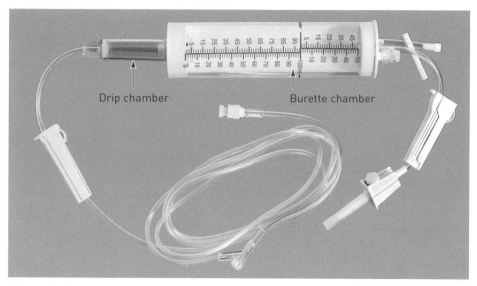

Figure 7.6 Administration set with micro-drop burette

Source: Wellcome Images

Calculate the following infusion rates in drops per minute if the fluid is to be given intravenously via a **micro-drop administration set** that delivers 60 drops per millilitre (correct to the nearest whole drop).

(d) 200 mL 0.9% saline over 2 hours = _____

(e) 150 mL 5% glucose over 1 hour 40 minutes = _____

(f) 250 mL sodium chloride 0.18% with 4% glucose over 3 hours = _____

Calculate the following infusion rates in drops per minute if the fluid is to be given intravenously via a blood administration set that delivers 15 drops per millilitre (correct to the nearest whole drop).

(g) 475 mL whole blood over 3 hours = _____

(h) 475 mL whole blood over 1.5 hours = _____

(i) 225 mL of packed cells over 4 hours = _____

Calculate the following infusion rates in mL/hour if the fluid is to be given intravenously via a volumetric pump (to the nearest millilitre).

(j) 1 L 0.9% saline over 6 hours = _____

(k) 500 mL 5% glucose over 2 hours = _____

(l) 500 mL of Ringer's solution over 3 hours = _____

Answers: (a) 56 dpm (b) 67 dpm (c) 83 dpm (d) 100 dpm (e) 15 dpm (f) 83 dpm (g) 40 dpm (h) 79 dpm (i) 14 dpm (j) 167 mL/hour (k) 250 mL/hour (l) 167 mL/hour.

If you had these all correct, well done. Now go to Section 7.2 for other delivery devices.

Drops per minute

If an infusion is being controlled manually, the rate is regulated by the roller clamp and by the height of the infusion fluid above the ground because the flow depends on **gravity**.

Look at the example prescription in Table 7.1 and identify the type and volume of fluid ordered. Over what period of time does it have to be given?

Here 1 litre of 0.9% sodium chloride is to be given over 6 hours but we want to give the fluid in drops per minute.

So how do we do that?

First find the number of drops that are in 1 L of fluid. It doesn't matter what fluid it is, the administration set will deliver the number of drops per millilitre that it says on the packet. The standard set gives 20 drops per mL (drops/mL).

There are 1000 mL in 1 litre and each millilitre contains 20 drops. You can now calculate how many drops there are in a litre – can't you?

$$1000 \, mL \times 20 \, drops \, mL = 20\,000 \, drops$$

You now need to find the number of minutes over which these drops have to be given. The prescription states that the fluid has to run over 6 hours, but you want minutes, so multiply the number of hours by 60 to make it into minutes:

$$6 \, hours \times 60 = 360 \, minutes$$

Now you have the information in the format needed, you just have to find the number of drops per minute by dividing the number of drops by the number of minutes:

$$\frac{20\,000}{360} = 55.55 \, drops \, per \, minute$$

You can't give part of a drop, so you correct the answer to the nearest whole number. In this case the answer is 56 drops per minute.

 If you need to revise calculating fractions, look at Chapter 2.

This must be as accurate as possible, so once you have checked your calculation, you need to use a watch with a seconds hand and count the drops as they pass through the drip chamber, adjusting the flow with the roller clamp until the rate is correct.

The rate needs to be checked after half an hour to make sure that it is still correct, adjusting if necessary.

The way in which this calculation has been done can be used to work out any infusion rate that is manually controlled as long as you know the drop delivery of the administration set, the volume of fluid in millilitres and the time, in minutes, over which it has to be given.

The formula to calculate the infusion rate in drops per minute is

$$\frac{\text{number of millilitres to be given} \times \text{drops per mL of the giving set}}{\text{number of hours} \times 60} = \text{drops per minute}$$

EXAMPLES

Calculate the drops per minute at which the following infusions should be set.

(a) A patient is to be given 500 mL of 5% dextrose over 4 hours, using a standard administration set.

Number of millilitres	500 mL
Number of minutes	4 × 60
Drops per millilitre	20

You don't need to change the volume since this is prescribed in millilitres, but it could also be written as 0.5 L so think before you calculate!

Now put the figure into the formula:

$$\frac{500 \times 20}{4 \times 60} = 41.66$$

$$= 42 \text{ drops per minute}$$

(rounded to the nearest whole number).

(b) A patient is to be given 50 mL of antibiotic over 1 hour using a micro-drop administration set.

Number of millilitres	50 mL
Number of minutes	1 × 60
Drops per millilitre	60

$$\frac{50 \times 60}{1 \times 60} = 50 \text{ drops per minute}$$

(c) A blood transfusion of 475 mL is to be given via a blood administration set over 3 hours.

Number of millilitres	475 mL
Number of minutes	3 × 60
Drops per millilitre	15

$$\frac{475 \times 15}{3 \times 60} = 39.58$$

$$= 40 \text{ drops per minute}$$

(rounded to the nearest whole number).

TIME TO TRY

Calculate the number of drops per minute (to the nearest whole drop) that the following infusions should be given if a standard infusion set is being used.

(a) 1 litre of 5% glucose over 4 hours = _____

(b) 500 mL of 0.9% sodium chloride over 2.5 hours = _____

(c) 250 mL of Ringer's solution over 2 hours = _____

Calculate the number of drops per minute (to the nearest whole drop) that the following infusions should be given if the administration set delivers 60 drops per millilitre.

(d) 100 mL 0.9% saline over 2 hours = _____

(e) 250 mL 5% glucose over 1 hour 40 minutes = _____

(f) 250 mL sodium chloride 0.18% and 4% glucose over 2 hours = _____

Calculate the number of drops per minute (to the nearest whole drop) that the following infusions should be given if the administration set delivers 15 drops per millilitre.

(g) 475 mL whole blood over 2 hours = _____

(h) 475 mL whole blood over 3.5 hours = _____

(i) 225 mL of packed cells over 4 hours = _____

Answers: (a) 83 dpm (b) 67 dpm (c) 42 dpm (d) 50 dpm (e) 150 dpm (f) 125 dpm (g) 59 dpm (h) 48 dpm (i) 14 dpm.

If you need more practice, there are further examples at the end of the chapter.

Millilitres per hour

Intravenous fluids contain additives which may cause adverse reactions if given too rapidly or some patients may be vulnerable to **fluid overload**. In these situations the fluid is given via a pump that delivers the fluid in millilitres per hour. The rate of fluid delivery needs to be calculated first and then entered into the panel.

If we use the prescription from Table 7.1 and use a volumetric pump (Figure 7.3) we need the volume of fluid in millilitres and the time in hours to calculate the millilitres per hour.

Millilitres   1000 mL
Hours   6

$$\frac{\text{millilitres}}{\text{hours}} = \frac{1000}{6} = 166.66 = 167 \text{ mL per hour}$$

(to the nearest whole millilitre).

TIME TO TRY

Calculate the following infusion rates in mL/hour if the fluid is to be given intravenously via a volumetric pump (to the nearest millilitre).

(a) 1 L of 0.9% saline over 4 hours = _____

(b) 0.5 L of 5% glucose over 2 hours = _____

(c) 500 mL of Ringer's solution over 4 hours = _____

Answers: (a) 250 mL/hour (b) 250 mL/hour (c) 125 mL/hour.

If you need more practice, there are further examples at the end of the chapter.

KEY POINTS

Intravenous infusions can be delivered through an infusion pump at a rate of millilitres per hour:

- Divide the prescribed volume in millilitres by the number of hours over which the fluid has to be given.

Manually regulated fluids are given using an administration set that drips a known number of drops per millilitre. The infusion is regulated to flow at drops per minute:

- The prescribed volume of fluid in millilitres is multiplied by the number of drops that the administration set delivers, to give the total number of drops.

- The hours over which the fluid has to run are multiplied by 60 to give the number of minutes.

- The number of drops is divided by the number of minutes to give the rate of delivery in drops per minute.

7.2 OTHER DRUG DELIVERY DEVICES

Patient-controlled analgesia (PCA)

Post-operative management of pain is important for early recovery. Pain is a subjective experience, so giving a patient control over the administration of pain relief helps to keep discomfort to a tolerable level.

You will find different models of PCA delivery systems. One type consists of a large syringe filled with the prescribed total amount of drug placed in a special **syringe pump** that is covered by a locked clear door. Another type of pump has the drug contained in a small infusion bag, as seen in **Figure 7.7**. An electrically operated push-button is controlled by the patient, to administer a predetermined dose of the drug to themselves.

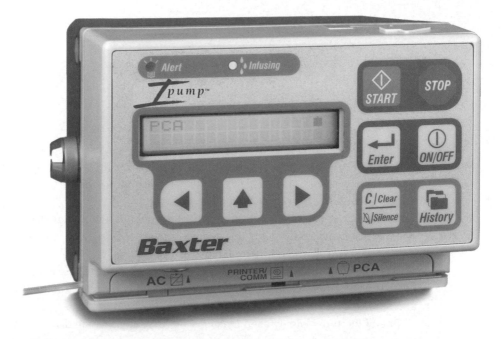

Figure 7.7 A patient-controlled analgesia (PCA) pump
Source: Baxter Healthcare Ltd

The maximum frequency and dose of the drug are set by the clinical staff so that the patient can't accidentally give themselves an overdose.

Many PCA devices have a downloadable memory log so that the total amount of drug used can be recorded and dosages adjusted if necessary.

Typically, a dose is calculated according to the patient's weight but in the case of morphine the patient's age is taken into account. This calculation is carried out by a trained member of staff, but if you are caring for the patient you need to monitor the patient and have some idea of how long the drug will last in order to alert someone to prepare more or review the regime.

EXAMPLE

A 30 mL syringe is filled with an analgesic drug such as morphine in a concentration 6 mg/mL. The patient is able to deliver 3 mg at a minimum interval of 10 minutes. If the patient uses a dose every 10 minutes, how long will the 30 mL syringe last?

First find the total amount of drug in the syringe:

$$30 \text{ mL} \times 6 \text{ mg/mL} = 180 \text{ mg}$$

$$\text{Then number of doses per hour} = \frac{60 \text{ min}}{10 \text{ min}} = 6$$

$$\text{mg/hour} = \text{number of doses/hour} \times \text{mg/dose}$$
$$= 6 \times 3 = 18 \text{ mg/hour}$$

137

There is 180 mg in total, so divide it by the number of mg/hour to find the time it will last:

$$\frac{180\,mg}{18\,mg/hour} = 10\,hours$$

Syringe drivers

The PCA pump limits the patient's mobility and may not be suitable for all patients who need a continuous level of analgesia, so a syringe driver is better as it is compact, battery driven and easily portable. The drugs are given through a special **subcutaneous** needle rather than intravenously.

Syringe drivers are used for a variety of drugs, not just analgesics. The syringe needs to be compatible with the syringe driver and, as with all the equipment described so far, comes in several types.

The merits of individual makes is not in question but the one used in a particular setting often depends on clinicians' choice and contract agreements for supply and servicing.

One of the most widely used makes is the Graseby syringe driver. There are two models: one that delivers drugs at an hourly rate and one that delivers the dose of drug over 24 hours. They look very much the same, but the 1 hour machine has a blue label and 1 h on its front and the 24 hour machine has a green label with 24 h in large numbers (**Figures 7.8 (a) and (b)**).

The dose of drug to be given via one of these syringes may be prescribed in different ways, so the person responsible for administration must work out the total dose to be given.

Format of the prescription

1. A dose is to be given every 3 hours (or any time interval). The first step is to calculate the total dose for 24 hours.

   For example, a patient is prescribed diamorphine 10 mg every 4 hours to be given via a syringe driver.

   Work out the number of times this dose would be given:

$$\frac{24\,hours}{4\,hours} = 6\,doses$$

   Now calculate the total amount of drug in 24 hours:

$$10\,mg \times 6 = 60\,mg$$

2. The dose is prescribed in milligrams per hour. Again the total dose for 24 hours has to be calculated.

   For example, a patient is prescribed a dose of diamorphine 5 mg per hour.

   Work out the dose for 24 hours:

$$5\,mg\ per\ hour\ for\ 24\ hours = 5\ mg \times 24\ hours = 120\ mg/24\ hours$$

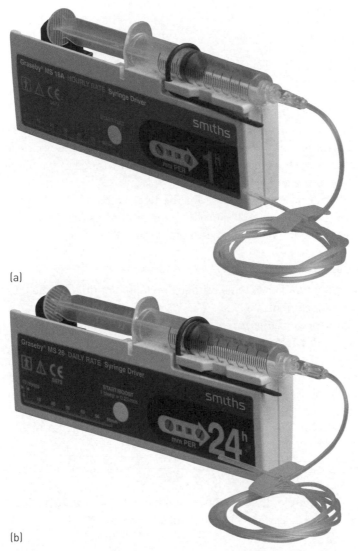

(a)

(b)

Figure 7.8 Graseby syringe drivers: (a) 1 hour MS 16A blue panel; (b) 24 hour MS 26 green panel

Source: Smiths Medical International

3. A prescription may also be written as a straightforward dose for 24 hours so there is no need for a further calculation.

   For example, a patient is prescribed diamorphine 80 mg for 24 hours.

4. A prescription may state a period of time of less than 24 hours.

   For example, a patient is prescribed diamorphine 15 mg to be given over 6 hours.

Setting up the syringe driver

Whichever make of syringe driver is used, the rate at which the machine is set does not rely on the actual volume of the drug in the syringe but on the length of the column of fluid.

139

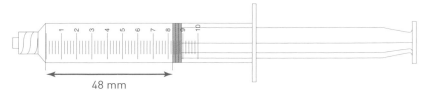

48 mm

Figure 7.9 Measuring the length of fluid in the syringe

The syringe driver has a millimetre scale on the edge of the front panel and can be used to measure the length of fluid from the upper edge of the plunger to the 0 line at the top of the syringe.

The amount of drug for 24 hours (or the total amount if less than 24 hours) is mixed with the appropriate diluting fluid, the volume is drawn into the specified type of syringe and the length is measured (**Figure 7.9**).

Setting the rate

If the connecting tubing has to be primed, the length of fluid will be less than if the syringe is a replacement.

Ideally the length of fluid should be divisible by 24, since this makes the arithmetic easier, if it is to be given over a 24-hour period.

If the length of fluid is 48 mm and the drug has to be given over 24 hours, then the calculation of the rate will be different whether the MS 16A (mm/hour) or the MS 26 (mm/24 hours) is used:

$$\text{MS 16A rate} = \frac{\text{length of fluid (mm)}}{\text{infusion time in hours}} = \text{rate in mm/hour}$$

$$\text{MS 26 rate} = \frac{\text{length of fluid (mm)}}{\text{infusion time in 24 hours (1 day)}} = \text{rate in mm/24 hours (1 day)}$$

The measured length of fluid is 48 mm and it has to be given over 24 hours. If this is put into an MS 16A syringe driver it needs to be run at

$$\text{rate} = \frac{48 \text{ mm}}{24 \text{ hours}} = 2 \text{ mm/hour}$$

If using an MS 26 model the rate is

$$\text{rate} = \frac{48 \text{ mm}}{1 \text{ day}} = 48 \text{ mm/24 hours}$$

The rate at which each machine is set is very different, although the patient will have the same dose in a 24-hour period.

The setting for these rates is shown in **Figure 7.10**. It is important to put 2 mm as 02 mm otherwise the reading will be 20 mm/hour.

If the prescription specifies a period of less than 24 hours, then the MS 16A machine is the one to choose.

The dose of drug is dissolved in a convenient volume of fluid and the length, measured in millimetres, is divided by the number of hours.

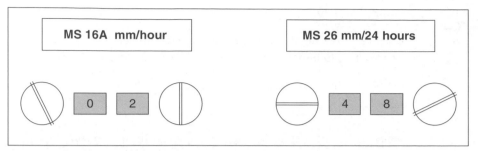

Figure 7.10 Setting the rate of flow on syringe drivers

For example, a patient is to receive diamorphine 10 mg over 6 hours:

$$\text{rate} = \frac{24\,\text{mm}}{6\,\text{hours}} = 4\,\text{mm/hour}$$

so the machine should be set at 04 mm/hour.

As you can see, there are a number of steps before the syringe driver can be connected to the patient, so it is better for two people to check the dilution, the length of fluid and the settings before pushing the start button.

KEY POINTS

Drugs given via a syringe driver need to be carefully prepared:

- Calculate the total dose to be given over 24 hours.
- Mix with appropriate fluid and make to a total volume that is easy to measure in multiples of 24.
- Measure the length of fluid in the barrel of the syringe in millimetres and then divide by 24 to give the hourly rate if using a syringe driver that delivers mm/hour (e.g. Graseby MS 16A).
- Divide the length of fluid by 24 hours (1 day) if using a syringe driver that delivers mm/24 hours (e.g. Graseby MS 26).
- Set the dials, making sure that a single number is preceded by a 0.

LOOK OUT

It is vital that you know which make and type of machine that is being used. Although you may not be responsible for setting up the equipment, if you are caring for a patient who is receiving this type of treatment then you should be aware of how to check that it is running satisfactorily.

You should also be aware that your clinical area may have specific guidelines about the management of syringe drivers, e.g. there may be a standard length of fluid that is recommended or only one model of equipment used.

TIME TO TRY

Calculate the rate at which the following lengths of diluted drug should be administered in (i) millimetres per hour and (ii) millimetres per 24 hours.

(a) 48 mm (i) = _____   (ii) = _____

(b) 24 mm (i) = _____   (ii) = _____

Answers: (a) (i) 02 mm/hour (ii) 48 mm/24 hours (b) (i) 1 mm/hour (ii) 24 mm/24 hours.

This book does not cover the all-important aspects of care and monitoring of the patient and the infusion site. You need to make yourself familiar with any local policies and procedures and read a clinically based textbook such as Dougherty and Lister (2008).

The risks of intravenous therapy are clearly highlighted by Ingram and Lavey (2005) and should give you food for thought.

> **RUNNING WORDS**
>
> | | | |
> |---|---|---|
> | burette | intravenous fluids | standard administration |
> | drops per minute | micro-drop | set |
> | fluid overload | administration set | subcutaneous |
> | gravity | patient-controlled | syringe driver |
> | intravenous (IV) | analgesia (PCA) | syringe pump |

Answers to the following questions can be found at the end of the book.

What did you learn?

(a) You need to select the appropriate fluid administration set to deliver 1 litre of 0.9% sodium chloride over a period of 6 hours. Which set would you choose and at what rate, in drops per minute, would you need to set the flow?

_____

_____

(b) A patient is to receive a blood transfusion of 450 mL to be given over a period of 4 hours. Which administration set would you choose and why? How many drops per minute should it be set at to transfuse the blood in the required time?

_____

_____

(c) Name four checks that should be taken when selecting a bag of intravenous fluid

_____

_____

(d) At what rate should 100 mL of fluid be given, in drops per minute, if it has to run over 30 minutes and if it is given

(i) with a standard administration set _____

(ii) a micro-drop burette set _____ ?

(e) A patient has a PCA pump that contains 30 mL of solution containing 4 mg/mL of morphine. A dose of 2 mg can be delivered on demand at an interval of every 10 minutes. If the patient presses the dose button five times each hour

(i) How much morphine will the patient have per hour? _____

(ii) How long will the 30 mL last if the patient has the same hourly dose?

_____

(f) How is the rate of flow measured when using a syringe driver? _____

(g) How do you calculate the rate of flow for a syringe driver that delivers an hourly amount of drug? _____

(h) How do you calculate the rate of flow for a syringe driver that delivers a 24 hour flow? _____

More 'Time to Try' examples

Page 135

Calculate the following infusion rate in drops per minute (dpm) if the fluid is to be given intravenously via a standard administration set that delivers 20 drops per millilitre (correct to the nearest whole drop).

(a) 500 mL of 10% glucose over 4 hours = _____

(b) 200 mL of Ringer's solution over 1 hour = _____

(c) 500 mL of sodium chloride 0.45% with 2.5% glucose over 3 hours = _____

Calculate the following infusion rates in drops per minute if the fluid is to be given intravenously via a micro-drop administration set that delivers 60 drops per millilitre (correct to the nearest whole drop).

(d) 250 mL 0.9% saline over 2 hours = _____

(e) 150 mL 5% glucose over 1 hour 30 minutes = _____

(f) 100 mL sodium chloride 0.18% with 4% glucose over 3 hours = _____

Calculate the following infusion rates in drops per minute if the fluid is to be given intravenously via a blood administration set that delivers 15 drops per millilitre (correct to the nearest whole drop).

(g) 475 mL whole blood over 4 hours = _____

(h) 475 mL whole blood over 2.5 hours = _____

(i) 225 mL of packed cells over 2 hours = _____

Page 136

Calculate the following infusion rates in mL/hour if the fluid is to be given intravenously via a volumetric pump (to the nearest mL).

(a) 1 L of 0.9% saline over 3 hours = _____

(b) 1000 mL of 5% glucose over 6 hours = _____

(c) 0.5 L of Ringer's solution over 2 hours = _____

Web resources

http://www.ismp.org/Newsletters/acutecare/articles/20030710.asp
Safety issues related to the use of patient-controlled analgesia.

www.nbt.nhs.uk/researcheducation/staff_development/calculations/
Further examples of drip rate calculations and some more advanced calculations for intravenous drug therapy.

http://www.medical-calculators.co.uk/driprate.html
You can make some of your own calculations and check the answers by putting them into this program.

http://www.epocrates.com/products/medtools/ivdripcalculator.html
You can download an infusion calculator onto a palm PDA.

References

Dougherty L. and Lister S. (2008) *The Royal Marsden Hospital Manual of Clinical Nursing Procedures*, 7th edn. Chichester: Wiley-Blackwell.

Ingram P. and Lavey I. (2005) Peripheral intravenous therapy: key risks and implications for practice. *Nursing Standard*, **19**(46): 55–64.

Chapter 8

Common clinical measurements

Charting, charting and more charting

A lot of your time will be spent in monitoring and recording vital signs, nutritional status and fluid balance. This chapter will help you to calculate and record these observations accurately.

When you have completed this chapter, you should be able to:

- Accurately chart recordings of vital signs.
- Calculate body mass index and body surface area.
- Take and record peak flow.
- Measure and record fluid intake and output.
- Screen patients for malnutrition.

Patients need to be monitored on a regular basis to detect any improvements or deterioration in their condition. You may hear the process being called 'doing the obs', a task that is often given to the most junior staff to undertake.

Major decisions can be taken on the results of these measurements, so it is vital that the person making the observations carries them out accurately and records them correctly and clearly. It is also a good opportunity to talk with the patient and get to know them, which will help in making an assessment of their condition.

Vital signs

Blood pressure, temperature, pulse and respiration rate are often taken at intervals during the day, the frequency being determined by the patient's condition. These are usually abbreviated to **TPR** and BP. Abbreviations are useful but it sometimes sounds as if the staff are speaking another language. When you have mastered those commonly used in one specialty, you will need to learn a new set when you move to another!

It is not the purpose of this book to describe in detail the taking of actual measurements but to look at the areas of accuracy of measurement and clarity of the recordings.

Unless the equipment is checked regularly in line with the manufacturer's instructions, then the recordings may be inaccurate. If you are using equipment, it is your responsibility to ensure that it is in working order, clean and appropriate to the patient's needs.

You need to be familiar with the paperwork associated with the recording of observations as there may be differences in the layout of the charts, though they will be showing the same parameters. An example of a vital signs chart is given in **Figure 8.1**.

There is a lot of information to take in when you look at charts, so take one section at a time to understand what is required for completion. The box in the top right corner must be completed clearly to ensure that loose documents can be matched together. If available, a printed label from the patient's records should be used. It is the responsibility of the trained nurse or doctor to order the frequency of the observations.

A list of some of the abbreviations in the chart and their meanings and translations can be found in Appendix E but for convenience these are freely translated here as: QDS, four times a day; TDS, three times a day; BD, twice daily; OD, daily.

LOOK OUT

A list of approved abbreviations should be available in the clinical area and others should not be used. Abbreviations can have different meanings in different care settings. In cardiology, AF is the abbreviation for atrial fibrillation, but in obstetrics means amniotic fluid.

Name	Date of Birth	Frequency of observations to be prescribed by registered nurse/medical staff.
Hospital Number	Date of Admission	Registered nurse to review observations each shift.
Ward	Consultant	Report readings if at level of < (less than) or > (more than)

	DATE	01.01.09				02.01.09				03.01.09				04.01.09				05.01.09				06.01.09				07.01.09				
		QDS	TDS	BD	OD	QDS	TDS	BD	OD	QDS	TDS	BD	OD	QDS	TDS	BD	OD	QDS	TDS	BD	OD	QDS	TDS	BD	OD	QDS	TDS	BD	OD	
	OTHER																													
	TIME	07:00	13:00	18.00	20.00	07:00	13:00	18.00	20.00	07:00	13:00	18.00	20.00	07:00	13:00	18.00	20.00	07:00	13:00	18.00	20.00	07:00	13:00	18.00	20.00	07:00	13:00	18.00	20.00	
Pulse Rate	>140																													>140
	140																													140
	130																													130
	120																													120
	110																													110
	>100																													>100
	90																													90
	80																													80
	70																													70
	<60																													<60
	50																													50
	40																													40
Blood Pressure mm Hg	220																													220
	210																													210
	200																													200
	190																													190
	180																													180
	170																													170
	>160																													>160
	150																													150
	140																													140
	130																													130
	120																													120
	110																													110
	100																													100
	<90																													<90
	80																													80
	70																													70
	60																													60
Respirations	>30																													>30
	25-29																													25-29
	20-24																													20-24
	15-19																													15-19
	10-14																													10-14
	<10																													<10
Temperature °C	39.0																													39.0
	38.8																													38.8
	38.6																													38.6
	38.4																													38.4
	38.2																													38.2
	38.0																													38.0
	37.8																													37.8
	37.6																													37.6
	37.4																													37.4
	37.2																													37.2
	37.0																													37.0
	36.8																													36.8
	36.6																													36.6
	36.4																													36.4
	36.2																													36.2
	36.0																													36.0
	Initials																													
	RN/HCA																													

Figure 8.1 City Hospital: temperature, pulse, respiration and blood pressure chart

Accurate charting

The information on any chart should be clear, accurate, complete and easy to read. **Figure 8.2** shows examples of different ways of entering the information. It is

147

clearer to use a cross (**X**) to identify the value of the observation, rather than the varying size of dot •.

Pulse, respiration and temperature observations should be linked together with straight lines. It is far easier to see at a glance how these rates fluctuate over a

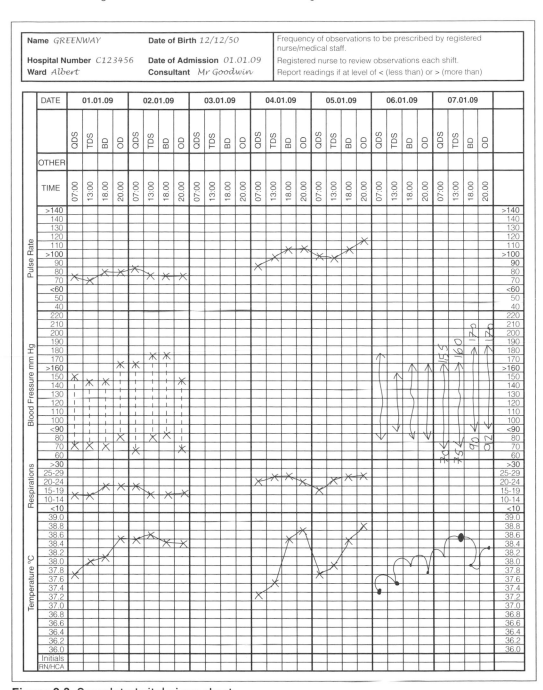

Figure 8.2 Completed vital signs chart

period of time. Curved lines joining the temperature recordings make reading the pattern difficult.

The arrowheads on the blood pressure readings do not indicate precisely into which band the number falls and the addition of numbers further confuses the issue. If exact recordings are needed for patients in intensive care, then more detailed charts are available with larger scales.

The patient information at the top of the chart is incomplete. All the details are needed to ensure that loose papers are filed in the correct set of patient documents.

APPLYING THE THEORY

Look at a patient's temperature chart and see if you can detect a pattern in the rise and fall over the course of a week. Patterns can give clues about some disease processes that have characteristic changes in the vital signs. Is it easy to read or are the lines curved so that you have difficulty in seeing a pattern?

8.1 PULSE, TEMPERATURE AND BLOOD PRESSURE

You will learn how the heart beats and generates a wave of blood through the elastic arteries causing them to stretch and recoil. The pulse can be found any-where an artery can be pressed against a bone. The most common site is the **radial artery**, near to the wrist.

When counting the pulse rate, you must start your count with 0, *not* 1, using the seconds hand on your watch to count for a *full* minute. Multiplying 15 seconds by 4 or 30 seconds by 2 or any other combination is not an accurate way to assess and record the pulse rate. When you are taking a pulse you also need to be thinking about the following:

● Is it regular or irregular?

● If it is irregular, is there a pattern to the irregularity or a random irregularity?

● Are the beats very strong or weak?

● Can you stop the blood flow by pressing gently on the artery?

● Does the artery feel soft or 'rubbery'?

A normal pulse rate for an adult at rest is 60–80 beats per minute. Children's pulse rate varies with age. Under 2s have a pulse of 90–130. Any abnormalities should be reported and recorded.

Adults with a pulse rate above 100 beats per minute are said to have **tachycardia**. Those with a rate below 60 beats per minute have **bradycardia**; however, athletes tend to have a slow pulse due to training.

A single reading is not useful for making a decision about a patient's condition. Vital signs vary with stress, exercise, food intake and age as well as illness. Measuring reg-ularly over a period of time will show trends up or down or regular fluctuations.

Table 8.1 Your pulse rate

TIME	At rest	After exercise	2 min	4 min	6 min	8 min	10 min	12 min	14 min	16 min	18 min	20 min
140												
140												
130												
120												
110												
>100												
90												
80												
70												
<60												
50												
40												

TIME TO TRY

Try taking your own pulse after you have been sitting down for at least 10 minutes. Make a note of the result in **Table 8.1**. Now jog on the spot for 5 minutes and take your pulse again and make a note. Sit and take your pulse at 2 minute intervals until it returns it to the resting level. How long did it take? Check your pulse when you are doing your normal activities and see how it changes. Compare the results with other students.

Now you should remember to check if any activities could affect the results when you measure a patient's vital signs.

Temperature

There are a number of types of equipment for measuring body temperature, but the mercury thermometer no longer features in the clinical areas because of the risks associated with mercury spillages from broken instruments.

In its place we have electronic thermometers that have a disposable sleeve (**Figure 8.3**) and that register the temperature in the mouth or **axilla** (under the arm). The temperature appears as a number in a window on the handle of the thermometer.

The other common method is to take the temperature next to the **tympanic membrane** (eardrum) using an infrared thermometer (**Figure 8.4**). To ensure that you obtain an accurate recording the tip must be close to the eardrum, so check the ears for wax and in the case of children for beads and Lego.

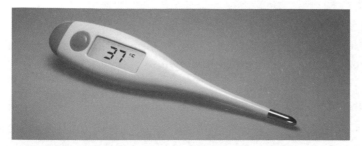

Figure 8.3 Electronic thermometer
Source: © Chris Collins/zefa/Corbis

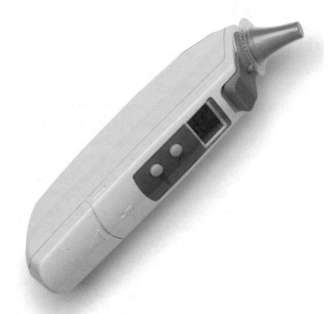

Figure 8.4 Infrared tympanic thermometer
Source: Mode Images Limited/Alamy

To get the tip close to the tympanic membrane, in an adult lift the ear *gently* upwards and backwards to straighten the ear canal. Children's ear canals need to be pulled *gently* downwards and slightly forwards. If you don't do these checks then the result will be inaccurate. The thermometer relies on taking the temperature of the blood flow at the bottom of the ear canal, which is close to the core temperature. A clean cover must be used for each patient.

The temperature is measured in degrees Celsius and is then recorded on the temperature chart.

The normal range of temperature is 36.6–37.2°C depending on the site from which it is recorded and the time of day. The temperature is towards the lower end of the range in the morning and at the higher end in the evening.

LOOK OUT

Make sure that you use a fresh cover tip for each patient for both types of thermometer to prevent **cross-infection**.

APPLYING THE THEORY

Patients with an infection or an inflammatory process may suffer a rise in temperature. It may also be accompanied by a rise in pulse rate. You also need to be aware that someone with a very severe infection may actually have a fall in temperature as the body starts to lose the fight. Older people tend to have a smaller rise in temperature than would be expected when they have an infection, whilst children can spike a frighteningly high temperature with an ear infection.

Blood pressure

Arterial walls contain elastic tissue which is able to stretch when under pressure from the extra blood pushed out when the ventricles of the heart contract. When the ventricles relax, the pressure falls. These two pressures vary with exercise, stress, age, elasticity of the arteries, circulatory volume and some disease processes.

The pressure in the arteries when the ventricles are contracting is known as the **systolic pressure** and the pressure when the ventricles are at rest is the **diastolic pressure**. The unit of pressure in SI is the pascal (Pa) but **millimetres of mercury (mmHg)** are used when measuring blood pressure because the size of the units is more convenient. Blood pressure is written as the systolic over the diastolic pressure, e.g. 120/80 mmHg. The difference between the two figures is called the pulse pressure, which in this case is 40 mmHg.

There has been a lot of publicity about the dangers of high blood pressure (**hypertension**), particularly the risk of heart attacks, kidney failure and strokes. People are more likely to be hypertensive if they smoke, don't take enough exercise or eat food high in salt and animal fat.

Not so much publicity is given to **hypotension** (low blood pressure), but this can be problematic since there will be a reduced amount of oxygen reaching the tissues. Hypotension follows a loss of blood or severe shock and is always a possibility after surgery, so patients need careful and frequent monitoring.

Blood pressure is measured using a **sphygmomanometer**. The equipment may be automated so that you only have to wrap the cuff around the patient's upper arm and the machine then inflates and deflates the cuff, giving a digital reading of the blood pressure (**Figure 8.5**).

Figure 8.6 is an example of a cuff. It is important to have the correct size in order to get an accurate reading. A wide cuff on a small arm will result in a lower reading than it should be and one that is too narrow on a large arm will result in a higher reading.

The accuracy of these machines has come into question and certainly they need at least weekly checks according to the manufacturer's guidelines.

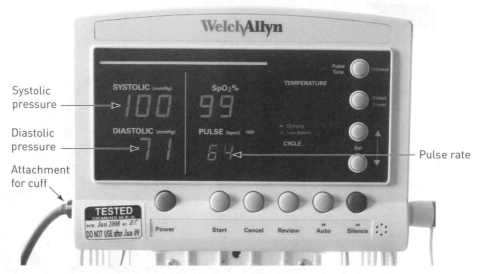

Systolic pressure

Diastolic pressure

Attachment for cuff

Pulse rate

Figure 8.5 An automated machine for recording blood pressure and pulse

Source: Mediscan

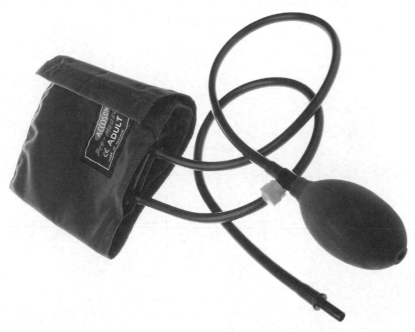

Figure 8.6 Blood pressure cuff

Source: Wellcome Images

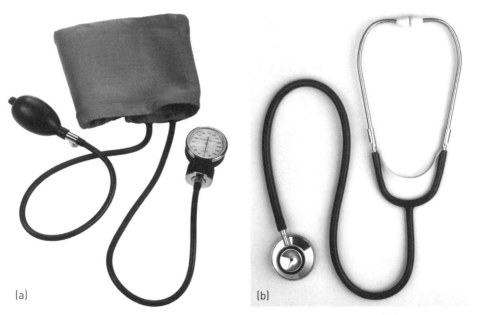

Figure 8.7 (a) Standard manual aneroid sphygmomanometer and (b) stethoscope

Source: (a) Geoff Kidd/Science Photo Library; (b) Gustoimages/Science Photo Library

Blood pressure can also be measured manually, using an aneroid sphygmo-manometer (**Figure 8.7**).

The cuff is placed around the patient's upper arm and inflated to stop the blood flow. Then you listen for the changes in the sound of the blood in the artery as you *slowly* let the air out of the cuff (**Figure 8.8**).

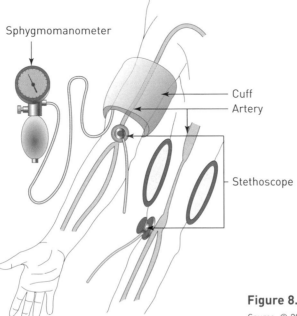

Sphygmomanometer

Cuff
Artery

Stethoscope

Figure 8.8 Measuring blood pressure

Source: © 2007 by Merck and Co., Inc.

The blood pressure reading is then entered into the chart making clear the upper and lower readings so that the pulse pressure can be seen easily. Details of how to take a recording can be found in a clinical skills textbook such as Docherty and Lister (2008).

8.2 RESPIRATORY MEASUREMENTS

We take breathing for granted until something goes wrong. It is the way oxygen is taken into the body and the waste carbon dioxide and water are removed. Our brain cells are very sensitive to oxygen levels and become irreversibly damaged if deprived of oxygen for more than 4 minutes. Respiratory rate is the least well documented of the vital signs.

Respiration is one parameter that can be controlled if the patient is aware of its being monitored. You should hold the patient's arm across their chest whilst taking the pulse. You can appear to still be taking their pulse but monitoring the respiration rate by counting the number of movements of the arm as the chest rises.

One respiration is a breath in (inspiration) and out (**expiration**) and should be counted for 1 minute. A normal range for an adult is 12–18 breaths per minute at rest, whilst the range for children varies with age, from 40+ for newborns to 25 for early teenagers.

As with the pulse, it is not just the rate of respiration that is of significance, but also depth of respiration, equal movement on both sides of the chest, any associated pain or difficulty with breathing known as **dyspnoea**. In dyspnoea, the patient may use their neck and shoulder muscles in an attempt to increase their air intake as well as puffing air out or blowing through almost closed lips. Also note any cough and sputum production.

APPLYING THE THEORY

Take the respiration rate of four of your colleagues. Compare the rates before and after exercise. What is the difference in the rate and the muscles used before and after exercise?

> ### KEY POINTS
> - The patient should be at rest before you measure vital signs.
> - Record rates for a whole minute, starting the count at 0.
> - Chart results immediately, using a cross to mark the point and join with straight line.
> - Report abnormalities immediately.

Other respiratory measurements

Think about your own breathing for a minute; most of the time you are breathing quietly in and out. The volume of air in and out is about 500 mL with each breath and is called the **tidal volume**. If your respiratory rate is 12 per minute, how many litres of air are moved in and out per minute?

Answer: 6 litres.

Now take the deepest breath in that you can and force as much air out as you are able as fast as you can.

This volume is about 3.5 L, depending on your size and gender. This volume is called the **forced vital capacity (FVC)**.

The rate at which air is moved out of the lungs is the **forced expiratory volume (FEV)**. Conditions such as asthma reduce this rate and air is retained in the lungs.

Patients with respiratory disease often have a reduced lung capacity. They are given medicines to alleviate the symptoms and it is useful to be able to find the lung volumes before treatment and monitor the effects. Some of the more complex tests are carried out in the respiratory laboratory, but some are straightforward enough to be carried out on the ward.

Peak expiratory flow rate (PEFR)

This is one of the tests that can be done on the ward or by the patient at home to monitor the efficacy of the treatment. This test measures the speed of the air coming out of the lungs, so any obstruction will slow the rate. The patient should have been resting before the test, and it can be carried out about half an hour after treatment.

The technique is to blow into the machine, a peak flow meter (**Figure 8.9**), as if blowing out a candle rather than blowing up a balloon. It is important to make sure that the patient understands what to do because they may not have enough breath for another go, although ideally the result should be the best of three attempts.

Lung volumes vary with height, age, gender and race. See Appendix G.

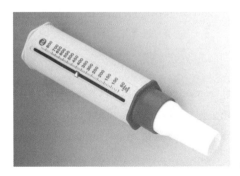

Figure 8.9 Wright's peak flow meter
Source: Clement Clarke International Ltd

Forced expiratory volume in 1 second (FEV₁)

As you saw earlier, the FVC involves getting as much air out as fast as possible, but the most important part is the amount of air in the first second. The technique for this test is to blow into the meter as if inflating a balloon as fast as possible.

The total volume expired is measured and then the percentage that was expired in the first second, the FEV_1. There are devices that can measure both PEFR and FEV_1 so that a more accurate assessment of lung function can be made.

There are a number of other measurements that can be carried out and if you have a patient booked for **spirometry**, try to find out about these tests.

Oxygen saturation

Oxygen is taken from the lungs to the tissues by the circulating red blood cells called **erythrocytes**. There is a limit to the amount of oxygen that can be carried in this way and we say that the cells are saturated with oxygen. When both the lungs and the red cells are functioning at their best, **oxygen saturation** is above 98%.

In areas where the blood flow is close to the surface, the oxygen saturation can be measured with a machine called a **pulse oximeter** (Figure 8.10). A wide clip is attached to the patient's finger, ear lobe or toe. Red light is produced in the clip and the amount of light passing through the tissue is measured and displayed as a percentage.

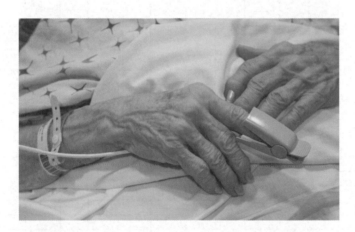

Figure 8.10 Pulse oximeter probe

Source: © Photographers Choice/Getty Images

> **LOOK OUT**
>
> Make sure that the patient's skin is not cold, because when the blood vessels constrict the reading will be inaccurate. If a patient is prescribed oxygen therapy, this will need to be noted on the observation chart where oxygen saturation is recorded.

8.3 FLUID BALANCE

As you saw in Chapter 7, maintaining a patient's fluid balance is vital to their well-being.

The volume of fluid lost from the body should be replaced by an equal volume of fluid – **fluid balance**. When a patient needs to have their intake and output measured, every drop of fluid taken into the body and all fluids leaving must be recorded on a 24-hour fluid balance chart like the one in **Figure 8.11**. As with all paperwork, each unit has one that meets its particular requirements so you need to familiarise yourself with the ones you will be using.

Mr/Mrs/Ms	Surname		Date	Over previous 72 hours		Balance
				Intake	Output	
First Name						
Date of Birth	Hospital No					
Ward	Consultant					

Date

Time	INTAKE in millilitres									OUTPUT in millilitres					
				IV 1			IV 2					Drainage 1		Drainage 2	
	Oral	Running total	Blood volume	Type	Vol.	Running total	Type	Vol.	Running total	Urine	Running total	Vol.	Running total	Vol.	Running total
01:00															
02:00															
03:00															
04:00															
05:00															
06:00															
07:00															
08:00															
09:00															
10:00															
11:00															
12:00															
13:00															
14:00															
15:00															
16:00															
17:00															
18:00															
19:00															
20:00															
21:00															
22:00															
23:00															
24:00															
Totals															

| Total Intake | millilitres | Total Output | millilitres |

Balance for today _____   Estimated insensible loss _____

Figure 8.11 Fluid balance chart

The fluids that are entered on the chart include:

Fluids intake

- Orally, including via a naso-gastric tube
- Intravenously
- Subcutaneously

Fluid output

- Urine
- Vomit
- Wound drainage
- Liquid faeces

Measuring intake

Oral intake

The volume of fluid contained in a disposable cup, plastic tumbler or china cup is different. It also depends on how full you make the container: plastic tumblers often have two sections, a ridged bottom part and a smooth band at the top. When pouring fluid into one of these you should be aware that there is almost as much volume above the ridges as there is below.

Some clinical areas will ask you to put in the type of fluid given, e.g. tea, squash, and may include jelly as fluid intake.

Oral intake also includes liquid feeds given via a naso-gastric tube or a tube inserted directly into the stomach.

Intravenous/subcutaneous

Patients who are unable to take in sufficient food or fluids orally may receive intravenous or subcutaneous fluids, which were discussed in Chapter 7. When the bag is started, the volume and type of fluid are entered into the correct column on the chart and the time noted when the bag is empty. Any volume left at the end of the 24-hour period is subtracted from the original volume and carried forward to the next day's chart and the volume given added to the current chart.

You can estimate the volume given/left from the scale on the side of the bag, but more accurately the bag can be weighed and the weight of the empty bag subtracted (1 mL of clear fluid weighs 1 g).

Measuring output

Urine

Disposable cardboard bedpans and urinals are used in many hospitals and it is easy to weigh the container when empty and then weigh it again after use; the difference in the weight in grams equals the volume in millilitres. Urine can also be transferred to a graduated jug to measure the volume.

Some patients need a catheter inserted into their bladder for one or more reasons and the output has to be recorded. How often the drainage bag is emptied varies, but the less frequently, the less risk of introducing infection; however, the output has to be measured at least every 24 hours.

Vomit and faeces

These are less pleasant to deal with but are far worse for the patient. The best method is to weigh them in the cardboard container to get a good approximation or to empty the container and refill it with the same amount of water.

Wound drainage

Valuable nutrients, as well as fluid, are lost through wound drainage so protein replacement, as well as fluid, needs to be considered. Wound drainage from recently made wounds is usually collected in a vacuum bottle which has a gauge on the side.

Chronic wounds are more of a problem since the wound drainage soaks into dressings. Some wound care specialist nurses suggest that the dressings are weighed before application and again after removal.

Insensible loss

Fluid is also lost in the form of perspiration and water vapour excreted during respiration. This is called **insensible loss**. Unless the patient is obviously sweating, insensible loss accounts for approximately 600–1000 mL per 24 hours and needs to be taken into account with the overall 24-hour fluid balance.

TIME TO TRY

(a) A cardboard bedpan weighs 47 g when empty. When a patient has passed urine, it weighs 439 g. What is the volume of urine that must be entered on the fluid balance chart? _____

(b) A cardboard urinal weighs 53 g when empty and 526 g after use. What volume of urine must be entered on the fluid balance chart? _____

Answers: (a) 392 mL (b) 473 mL.

How does it all add up?

Each drink that the patient has is entered onto the chart in the appropriate box and in the case of **Figure 8.11** is added to the previous amount, to give a running total. This makes it easier to complete at the end of the day, but not all fluid charts are in this format.

At the end of the 24-hour period, the totals for each column of fluid in and fluid out are written in the boxes at the bottom of the chart. The totals of the intake columns are added together and those of all the outputs are added together.

The output total is subtracted from the intake total and the balance recorded.

If there is a greater intake than output, it is recorded as a positive balance but if less than output it is a negative balance. In Figure 8.11 there is a space at the top to summarise the previous 3 days' balance, which is useful since it is difficult to make a decision about treatment on one set of observations.

Some patients have a restricted fluid intake because of kidney disease and their intake for any 24-hour period is calculated on insensible loss of 1 L plus a volume equal to the previous day's urinary output.

Patients who are given drugs to increase their urinary output (**diuretics**) will be expected to have a negative balance. Another way of measuring fluid loss is to weigh the patient accurately. How much does a litre of water weigh?

An example of a completed fluid balance chart is shown in **Figure 8.12**.

Mr/Mrs/Ms	Surname *GREENWAY*	Date	Over previous 72 hours		Balance
			Intake	Output	
First Name *Amanda*		*New admission*			
Date of Birth *12/12/50*	Hospital No *C123456*				
Ward *Albert*	Consultant *Mr GOODWIN*				

Date *01/01/09*

Time	INTAKE in millilitres									OUTPUT in millilitres					
				IV 1			IV 2					Drainage 1 VOMIT		Drainage 2	
	Oral	Running total	Blood volume	Type	Vol.	Running total	Type	Vol.	Running total	Urine	Running total	Vol.	Running total	Vol.	Running total
01:00															
02:00															
03:00															
04:00															
05:00															
06:00															
07:00				N/S	1000										
08:00										300	300				
09:00	100	100													
10:00															
11:00	100	200		5% D	1000	1000									
12:00										550	850				
13:00															
14:00	150	350										420	420		
15:00															
16:00										450	1300				
17:00	100	450							2000						
18:00															
19:00												150	570		
20:00	150	600													
21:00										200	1500				
22:00															
23:00															
24:00															
Totals		600				2000					1500		570		

| Total Intake | 2600 | millilitres | Total Output | 2070 | millilitres |

Balance for today *+ 530 mL*   Estimated insensible loss *600 mL*

Figure 8.12 Completed fluid balance chart

> **KEY POINTS**
> - Make sure that you know the amount of fluid held by each type of cup or glass.
> - Remember to complete chart after measuring output.
> - Take insensible loss into account when completing the fluid balance chart.

TIME TO TRY

A male patient has two cups of tea with his breakfast at 08:00, a cup of coffee at 10:00, a glass of squash at 11:00, a bowl of soup at lunchtime, a glass of water at 14:00, another cup of tea at 15:00, a glass of squash at 17:00, coffee at 18:00, a cup of hot chocolate at 20:00 and a glass of squash at 22:00.

He passes 455 mL of urine at 06:00, 400 mL at 10:30, 390 mL at 15:00, 320 mL at 20.00 and 300 mL at 22:30.

If a cup holds 130 mL, a glass 150 mL and a soup bowl 250 mL, what is his fluid balance, excluding insensible loss?

Answer: Negative balance of 235 mL.

There are more examples at the end of the chapter.

8.4 WEIGHT, HEIGHT AND NUTRITION

There have been many articles written highlighting the poor nutritional intake of patients in hospital, particularly the elderly. In the general population, the main areas of concern are the extremes of malnutrition – obesity and underweight individuals, especially amongst the young. Both extremes of the malnutrition scale are detrimental to health and long-term well-being.

Height and weight

These measurements are basic to assessing the physical state of a patient.

There have been some reports about the accuracy of hospital scales, with some patients being given the wrong amount of drug because the scales had not been correctly maintained. Accuracy of weight estimation is also important when monitoring the effects of a weight gaining or reducing diet as well as calculating the dose of drugs that are given according to weight.

Height should be recorded with the patient standing without shoes. If the patient is unable to stand and not sure of their height, the length of the **ulna** should be measured from the point of the elbow to the wrist. Tables are available to translate this into an approximate height, depending on gender and age (see the BAPEN website). If you are a Patricia Cornwell or Kathy Reichs fan then you will be familiar with measuring the bones of a skeleton to estimate height and age.

Height and weight are used to calculate **body surface area** and body mass index.

Body surface area

Some drugs, as you saw in Chapter 4, are given according to body surface area.

The surface area is the amount of skin covering the body. An adult 1.7 m tall and weighing 70 kg has a surface area of 1.8 m². If you can't imagine how much that is, it is approximately 24 sheets of A4 paper! There are charts, called nomograms, which allow you to calculate the body surface area using the height and weight of the patient. See Appendix I.

The body surface area can also be calculated using the following formula if you do not have a chart:

$$\text{body surface area} = \sqrt{\frac{\text{height in centimetres} \times \text{weight in kg}}{3600}}$$

EXAMPLE

To find the body surface area of a patient who is 1.5 m tall and weighs 65 kg, first put the figures into the above equation and work out the fraction in brackets, using a calculator:

$$\frac{150 \times 65}{3600} = \frac{9750}{3600} = 2.7$$

Now press the square root key ($\sqrt{\ }$) on the calculator, followed by the = sign:

$$\sqrt{2.7} = 1.63 \text{ m}^2$$

TIME TO TRY

Calculate the body surface area, correct to one decimal place, for patients with the following height and weight.

(a) Height 1.9 m, weight 64 kg, BSA = _____ m²

(b) Height 1.6 m, weight 59 kg, BSA = _____ m²

(c) Height 1.75 m, weight 119 kg, BSA = _____ m²

(d) Height 1.40 m, weight 62 kg, BSA = _____ m²

Answers: (a) 1.8 m² (b) 1.6 m² (c) 2.4 m² (d) 1.6 m²

There are more examples at the end of the chapter.

Body mass index (BMI)

A person's **BMI** is used as a broad assessment of whether or not the relationship between their weight and height is within a healthy range. A high BMI is associated with an increased risk of cardiovascular disease. This estimate is only suitable for adults.

You first need to measure the patient's height in metres and weight in kilograms. The weight is then divided by the height squared:

$$\text{BMI} = \frac{\text{weight in kg}}{\text{height in m}^2}$$

EXAMPLE

For a patient who is 1.8 m tall and weighs 70 kg

$$\text{BMI} = \frac{70}{1.6 \times 1.6} = \frac{70}{2.56} = 27.34 = 27$$

(to the nearest whole number).

There are a number of tables available that do the calculation and show the band into which the BMI falls. See Appendix H.

Range of BMI

Underweight	less than 20
Ideal weight	20 up to 25
Overweight	25 up to 30
Obese	30 up to 40
Very obese	over 40

TIME TO TRY

Calculate the BMI, to the nearest whole number, using the following information and identify in which range it falls.

(a) Height 1.9 m, weight 64 kg, BMI = _____, range = _____
(b) Height 1.6 m, weight 59 kg, BMI = _____, range = _____
(c) Height 1.73 m, weight 119 kg, BMI = _____, range = _____
(d) Height 1.4 m, weight 62 kg, BMI = _____, range = _____
(e) Height 1.55 m, weight 67 kg, BMI = _____, range = _____

Answers: (a) 18, underweight (b) 23, normal (c) 40, very obese (d) 32, obese (e) 28, overweight.

More examples can be found at the end of the chapter.

A rough estimate of BMI can be made by measuring the mid-arm circumference of the upper arm. Details of this assessment can be found at the BAPEN website, as can a chart for calculating BMI using the patient's weight and height.

APPLYING THE THEORY

Think about how you can judge whether someone has recently lost or gained weight.

Some things that you might notice are loose clothing, a change in the hole used on a belt, dull brittle hair, or poor skin condition with weight loss or tight clothing if there is weight gain.

Try to estimate a patient's height and weight before actually measuring them. It is good practice for times when you may not have scales and a tape measure to hand.

> **KEY POINTS**
> - Body mass index (BMI) is the relationship between height and weight.
>
> - $BMI = \dfrac{\text{weight in kg}}{\text{height in m}^2}$
>
> - Body surface area (BSA) varies with weight and height and can be calculated with a **nomogram** or by finding the square root of
>
> $\dfrac{(\text{height in centimetres} \times \text{weight in kg})}{3600}$.

Malnutrition universal screening tool (MUST)

The problem of malnutrition of patients in both hospitals and the community raised so much concern that a search was made for a screening tool that would identify most patients at risk. The 'Malnutrition Universal Screening Tool (MUST)' is an assessment that has been adopted by many hospital and community trusts.

It is useful because it is easy to carry out an assessment of the risk of malnutrition and gives guidelines for the management of the patient.

Patients scoring 0 are low risk, a score of 1 is medium risk and high risk if they score 2–6. The assessment recommends that all hospital patients are reviewed weekly regardless of their score and appropriate nutritional support given.

The full assessment document can be found on the BAPEN website.

Nutritional intake

When people are ill, the rate at which they use **energy** is often *increased* due to

- Fever
- Metabolic response to trauma
- Metabolic needs to repair tissue damage
- Sepsis.

Or they may have a *loss* of nutrients due to:

- Wound drainage
- Severe haemorrhage
- Kidney disease
- Diarrhoea and vomiting.

Or they may not be digesting or absorbing nutrients due to:

● Reduced absorptive surface in the intestines

● Lack of enzymes to break the food down.

Elderly patients and those with respiratory disease often get exhausted by the process of eating and so do not take in sufficient energy.

Measuring energy

In SI, energy in food is measured in kilojoules (kJ). You are probably more familiar with calories, a term in all the popular magazines when they are persuading you that the latest diet will make you a size 0 in 2 weeks.

Calories are more correctly called kilocalories (kcal): 1 kcal is approximately equivalent to 4.2 kJ. If you look at the table of nutrients on the side of food packaging, you will see that the energy value is usually in both kilojoules and calories.

Food intake and energy use are rather like a bank account (see **Table 8.2**): if you put in more than you use, you will accumulate savings. Unfortunately, these savings are in the form of fat. If you use more than you pay in, then there will be a deficit, leading to weight loss.

Each gram of carbohydrate and protein produces 19 kJ (4.5 kcal) and 1 g of fat produces 38 kJ (9 kcal). As you can see, fat contains twice the energy of carbohydrate and protein.

Excess intake of carbohydrate or fat is stored in the body as fat but excess protein is removed from the body via the kidneys. This is the principle underlying the Atkins diet, which contains a high proportion of protein but is dangerous if the individual has reduced kidney function.

Table 8.2 Guidelines for the daily intake of major food groups

	Women	Men	Children 5–10 years
Energy	8400 kJ (2000 kcal)	10 500 kJ (2500 kcal)	7560 kJ (1800 kcal)
Protein	45 g	55 g	24 g
Carbohydrate	230 g	300 g	220 g
Fat	70 g	95 g	70 g

APPLYING THE THEORY

You need to be aware of patients who may need to make up deficits in the nutritional intake.

A patient has had surgery and is allowed only sips of water for the rest of the day but is given an intravenous infusion of 1 L 5% w/v dextrose over 8 hours. What is the patient's energy intake for the day?

Where do you start?

You need to know that dextrose is pure carbohydrate so it will have an energy value of 19 kJ per gram. How many grams of dextrose are there in the litre of 5% w/v dextrose?

 If you need a reminder of how to do this calculation go back to Chapter 6.

There are 50 g of dextrose in this solution. Each gram is 19 kJ (4.5 kcal) so the total energy value is

$$50 \times 19 \text{ kJ} = 950 \text{ kJ} \quad \text{or} \quad 50 \times 4.5 \text{ kcal} = 225 \text{ kcal}$$

Not exactly a feast! This patient will need careful assessment to ensure that the energy needs are met. If a patient does not feel like eating very much, then you need to make every mouthful count. Foods normally given a wide berth will add calories with little effort. Full-cream ice cream, chocolate, cream cakes, biscuits and butter and cream should be added to other food where possible. These are probably more tempting than the milky thickened drinks that are often on offer.

Serving small helpings may encourage a patient to eat. Food from the hospital kitchen is usually served in standard portions, so find a smaller plate and transfer a more manageable amount. Your patient may even ask for more!

LOOK OUT
When the ward is busy, this is the most important time to check that your patient's nutritional needs are met. It is not unknown for food to be left out of reach or patients not helped to manage their meal, so trays are cleared and the food has not been touched. Don't let it happen.

KEY POINTS
- Patients need to have their nutritional status assessed on admission and reviewed weekly if in hospital.
- Disease processes increase energy requirements.
- Food should be high in energy and given in small appetising portions.
- Be aware of patients who need help with eating and drinking.

TIME TO TRY
Just so that you are aware of how you can best add energy to a patient's diet, find the energy value of the following foods and what a portion looks like. The energy values vary slightly, depending on which make of product is used.

What is the energy content per 50 mL of the following?

(a) whole milk _____ kJ

(b) skimmed milk _____ kJ

(c) double cream _____ kJ

What is the energy value of 10 g of the following?

(d) strawberry jam _____ kJ

(e) butter _____ kJ

(f) soft margarine _____ kJ

(g) white sugar _____ kJ

(h) peanut butter _____ kJ

(i) honey _____ kJ

What is the energy value of 30 g of the following?

(j) cream cheese _____ kJ

(k) Cheddar cheese _____ kJ

(l) milk chocolate _____ kJ

Answers: (a) 136 kJ (b) 73 kJ (c) 990 kJ (d) 108 kJ (e) 305 kJ (f) 300 kJ (g) 160 kJ (h) 250 kJ (i) 132 kJ (j) 423 kJ (k) 507 kJ (l) 660 kJ.

RUNNING WORDS

axilla	expiration	oxygen saturation
blood pressure	forced expiratory	pulse oximeter
BMI	volume (FEV$_1$)	radial artery
body surface area	fluid balance	sphygmomanometer
bradycardia	forced vital capacity	spirometry
cross-infection	(FVC)	systolic pressure
diastolic pressure	hypertension	tachycardia
diuretic	hypotension	tidal volume
dyspnoea	insensible loss	TPR
energy	mmHg	tympanic membrane
erythrocyte	nomogram	ulna

Answers to the following questions can be found at the end of book.

What did you learn?

(a) What is the normal range of pulse rate at rest? _____

(b) If you recorded a patient's blood pressure as 130/70, which number is the diastolic pressure? _____

(c) Does the systolic pressure represent the pressure when the ventricles have relaxed or contracted? _____

(d) What do the following abbreviations mean?

   (i) TDS _____   (ii) OD _____

(e) How much fluid will be carried over if a patient has a litre of intravenous fluid starting at 22:00 and has to run over 8 hours? _____ mL

(f) A patient weighs 76 kg and is 1.85 m tall. Calculate:

   (i) their BMI _____   (ii) body surface area _____ m^2

(g) Name two disease processes that can increase the need for energy intake.

   (i) _____   (ii) _____

(h) What are the daily energy requirements for

   (i) a woman _____ kJ   (ii) a man _____ kJ?

More 'Time to Try' examples

Page 162

A patient had an operation and has an intravenous infusion of 1 L 5% w/v dextrose which started at 08:00 and ran for 6 hours. This was followed by 1 L of 0.9% w/v saline over 6 hours and then 1 L 5% w/v dextrose over 8 hours. The patient was allowed to start oral fluids at 15:00 with 30 mL water and had a further total of 200 mL of water in small amounts until midnight. At 23:30 the patient felt nauseated and vomited 300 mL. The urinary catheter bag was emptied at 14:00 and 690 mL recorded. When the bag was emptied at midnight there was a further 975 mL.

What is the patient's fluid balance for the day, assuming that the intravenous fluid regime ran to plan, and what volume of IV fluid is to be carried over to the next day?

Page 163

Calculate the body surface area, correct to one decimal place, for patients with the following height and weight.

(a) Height 0.9 m, weight 16 kg, BSA = _____ m^2

(b) Height 1.58 m, weight 70 kg, BSA = _____ m^2

(c) Height 2.2 m, weight 95 kg, BSA = _____ m^2

(d) Height 1.73 m, weight 82 kg BSA = _____ m^2

Page 164

Calculate the BMI using the following information and identify in which range it falls, to the nearest whole number:

(a) Height 1.4 m, weight 38 kg, BMI = _____, range = _____

(b) Height 1.6 m, weight 88 kg, BMI = _____, range = _____

(c) Height 1.9 m, weight 120 kg, BMI = _____, range = _____

(d) Height 1.65 m, weight 73 kg, BMI = _____, range = _____

(e) Height 1.5 m, weight 58 kg, BMI = _____, range = _____

Web resources

http://www.patient.co.uk/showdoc/40001830/
This is a detailed article on the measurement of the pulse and the significance of abnormalities. Useful reminder when you are tempted to sloppy habits!

http://www.pennhealth.com/health_info/animationplayer/heartbeat.html
Animation of blood flow through the heart.

http://a1977.g.akamai.net/f/1977/1448/1d/webmd.download.akamai.com/1448/Anatom-E-Tools/Heart/Heart_Tool.swf
Animation of normal and abnormal heartbeats.

http://www.pennhealth.com/health_info/animationplayer/blood_pressure.html
Animation of how blood pressure is produced.

http://www.pennhealth.com/health_info/animationplayer/breathing.html
Animation of breathing.

http://www.bapen.org.uk
Detailed MUST nutritional assessment tool. This site also includes a BMI calculation chart, measuring mid-arm circumference and ulnar length to calculate BMI in patients who can't be weighed or measured.

http://www.bmi-calculator.net/bmr-calculator/
Automatic calculation of BMI using height and weight input.

http://www.micromedical.co.uk/services/knowledge/spiro.asp
Description of how spirometry is carried out.

http://www.lacors.gov.uk/lacors/NewsArticleDetails.aspx?id=18737
Comment from Local Authorities Co-ordinators of Regulatory Services on the accuracy of hospital scales.

http://www.weightloss.com.au/food-tables.html
This site is very useful for finding out the energy value of almost any foodstuff. It also shows the mineral and vitamin content of the foods. Just click on the initial letter of the substance you need. There are a number of combinations of nutrients for each food but each list contains the energy value in both calories and kilojoules.

Suggested reading

Doherty L. and Lister S. (2008) *The Royal Marsden Manual of Clinical Nursing Procedures.* Chichester: Wiley-Blackwell.

Chapter 9

Physiological measurements

Blood, but no sweat and tears

The more you are able to recognise the normal physiological values and understand their significance, the earlier you will be able to recognise when your patient's condition is changing and to alert more experienced staff.

When you have completed this chapter, you should be able to:

- Identify normal haematological values.

- Recognise the normal range of biochemical values.

- Understand the significance of blood gas monitoring.

- Demonstrate an understanding of the importance of basal metabolic rate.

- Understand the significance of urine testing.

The purpose of this chapter is to introduce you to some of the common tests that are carried out to assist with diagnosis and monitor treatment. A good anatomy and physiology textbook will give you more detail of how these parameters are maintained (e.g. Marieb and Hoehn, 2007).

9.1 BLOOD

The body is kept healthy by all the systems being maintained in a state of balance. This is known as **homeostasis**. You saw in Chapter 8 how there are normal ranges of vital signs and so it is with other aspects of physiology.

Blood is one of the most important body fluids and samples can be used to determine whether or not the body is in a state of health. Blood has a solid portion in the form of **platelets** and red and white blood cells. The liquid portion is called the **plasma**; it makes up about 55% of the blood volume and contains dissolved salts (**electrolytes**), proteins such as **albumen** and those that are involved in blood clotting.

Cells and solids in action

Red blood cells, more properly called **erythrocytes**, contain haemoglobin which in its turn contains iron. Iron is important for carrying oxygen from the lungs to the cells of the body. The erythrocytes also pick up waste carbon dioxide from the cells and take it back to the lungs to be excreted.

Women tend to have a lower **haemoglobin** level than men mainly due to menstrual loss.

In anaemia there is a reduction in the oxygen-carrying power of the blood. Since it is the erythrocytes that are responsible for this function, they become the prime suspects in this event (**Table 9.1**).

A blood sample is taken and sent to the laboratory, where it is examined for the number, size (volume) and haemoglobin content of the cells as well as the overall amount of haemoglobin in a litre of whole blood. Any changes in any of these can produce anaemia. The number of immature cells, **reticulocytes**, is counted. The study of this aspect of the blood is called **haematology**.

TIME TO TRY

Use the information you learned in Chapter 3 to work out the following. The answers will help you to appreciate how small cells are.

(a) What decimal fraction of a gram is a picogram (pg)? _____

(b) Write out the number off erythrocytes, 5.5×10^{12} L, in full: _____ cells per litre

(c) The volume of a single red cell is 80 fL. What vulgar fraction of a litre is a femtolitre? _____ L

Table 9.1 Reference values for erythrocyte indices and causes of increase or decrease

Index	Normal range	Increase	Decrease
Red cell count (RCC/ RBC) Female Male	$3.9-5.5 \times 10^{12}$ L $4.5-6.2 \times 10^{12}$ L	Dehydration Congestive cardiac failure	Blood loss Iron deficiency anaemia
Reticulocyte count	$25-85 \times 10^9$ (0.2–2% of red cell count)	Vit. B_{12} deficiency Haemorrhage	Chronic infection Alcoholism
Haemoglobin (Hb) Female Male	120–160 g/L 130–175 g/L	Burns Dehydration	Haemorrhage Liver disease
Haematocrit or packed cell volume (PCV) Female Male	37–48% 0.37–0.48 L/L 41–52% 0.41–0.52 L/L	Dehydration Burns Shock	Pregnancy Anaemia
Mean cell volume (MCV)	80–95 fL	Chronic liver disease Alcohol abuse	Lead poisoning Rheumatoid arthritis
Mean cell haemo-globin (MCH)	28–35 pg/cell	See haemoglobin	See haemoglobin
Platelets (thrombocytes)	$150-350 \times 10^9$	Trauma Cirrhosis	Clostridial infection Radiation

(d) The haematology report for Mr Kennedy shows that his haemoglobin is 115 g/L. Is this within the normal range? _____

Proteins in the blood

The plasma proteins, especially albumen, help to keep fluid in the circulation. If they drop because of loss or due to poor nutrition, fluid leaks out and produces swelling, called oedema. You may have seen pictures of malnourished children who have pot bellies and swollen ankles whilst the other parts of their little bodies are just skin and bone. This swelling is oedema due to protein deficiency.

Clotting

Leaks in the system must be stopped and so the blood has a self-preservation system built in. The blood proteins **fibrinogen** and **prothrombin** are inactive until stimulated into action when there is damage to the tissues. When clotting takes place, the clotting factors from the plasma solidify, leaving serum.

Unfortunately this system is also activated when there is damage to the inside of blood vessels and clots will form, blocking off the blood supply in vital areas such as the heart or brain.

If a patient is at increased risk of clot formation, that patient will need drugs to reduce the clotting activity. Patients often refer to these drugs as 'blood thinners' but they should be called **anticoagulants**.

Two common anticoagulants are warfarin, which is given orally, and heparin, which you met in Chapter 5, given as a subcutaneous injection. You may have heard of warfarin being given as a rat poison where its job is to overdose the rat and cause it to bleed to death. Fortunately or unfortunately, according to your point of view, we now have a breed of super rats that thrive on a warfarin diet.

Warfarin is a powerful drug that interferes with another substance crucial to clot formation, vitamin K. A patient's blood must be monitored to get the right dose of the drug for a balance between clotting and bleeding.

Prothrombin time (PT) and International normalised ratio (INR)

There is such a wide variation in the way in which prothrombin time is reported anywhere between 8 and 20 seconds that it has now been overtaken by INR as the reference point for treatment. It is recommended that an INR of between 2.0 and 3.0 should be maintained when on treatment or for prevention (prophylaxis) of clot formation. The test should be carried out every 3 days at the start of the treatment, weekly and monthly when a steady level is reached. There are monitoring devices for patients to carry out their own tests in between hospital visits.

> **LOOK OUT**
>
> Patients who are taking anticoagulants need to be monitored for early signs of bleeding. Some of the signs that you should be looking for are bleeding gums, bruising and traces of blood in the urine.

White blood cells

There are several types of white blood cells in the circulation but there are far fewer than red cells per litre of blood. White cells, in general, are there to fight infection and attack foreign particles. There are approximately $4.5-10.5 \times 10^9$ per litre in total. When blood is taken for a white cell count, a count of each type of cell is usually requested, and a calculation of the percentage of each, called a **differential count**, is made. **Table 9.2** shows the absolute differential count and a few of the possible causes of abnormalities.

Table 9.2 Differential white count and causes of increase and decrease

Type of white cell	Normal range/L(%)	Increase	Decrease
Neutrophils	$2.7-7.5 \times 10^9$ (45–75)	Acute infections Gout	Septicaemia Anorexia nervosa
Basophils	$0-0.2 \times 10^9$ (0–2)	Chronic sinusitis Splenectomy	Shock Pregnancy
Eosinophils	$0-0.5 \times 10^9$ (0–6)	Allergic conditions Rheumatoid arthritis	Severe infection Cushing's syndrome
Lymphocytes	$1.5-4.5 \times 10^9$ (20–45)	Crohn's disease Toxoplasmosis	Renal failure AIDS
Monocytes	$0.2-0.8 \times 10^9$ (2–10)	Tuberculosis Brucellosis	Severe infection Severe stress

The accuracy of results is important, so if you are with the patient when blood is being collected make sure that:

● The patient is warm to help the blood flow.

● The tourniquet is not on for more than a minute, otherwise the sample will be concentrated.

● The sample is not shaken but mixed by gentle rolling.

● The specimen is labelled with the patient's details and put in the bag attached to the blood form.

● If you use a pre-printed label for the form, a label is put on the copies as well.

● The specimen reaches the laboratory as soon as possible.

Fantastic fluid

The liquid part of the blood, plasma, consists mainly of water and is a biological soup of dissolved salts, nutrients, waste products and hormones. Many of these substances hitch a ride on the protein molecules in the plasma.

The rich mixture of the blood (**Figure 9.1**) makes it an ideal medium for examining the physiological changes that take place during illness and disease. The concentration of ions (electrolytes) in the blood closely reflects the concentrations in the fluid surrounding the cells (**interstitial fluid**). Some of the normal ranges of ions are given in **Table 9.3**. A fuller list of reference values can be found in Appendix D.

Organic substances

Organic substances are complex molecules that contain carbon; glucose, for example. Some of the common organic compounds and their normal values are given in **Table 9.4**. Urea is sometimes referred to as blood urea nitrogen (BUN).

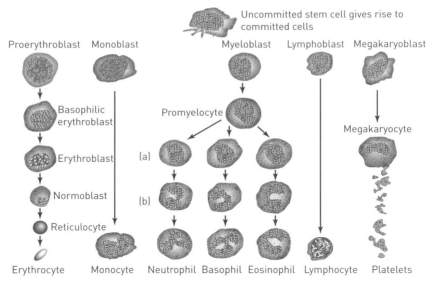

Figure 9.1 The different types of blood cells

Source: http://greenfield.fortunecity.com/rattler/46/haemopoiesis.htm © John Ross

Table 9.3 Normal ranges for ions in the plasma and causes of increase and decrease

Ion	Concentration	Increased	Decreased
Calcium (Ca^{2+})	2.1–2.6 mmol/L	Vitamin D excess Hyperparathyroidism	Rickets Diarrhoea
Chloride (Cl^-)	100–108 mmol/L	Kidney failure Dehydration	Burns Vomiting
Potassium (K^+)	3.6–5.0 mmol/L	Diabetic acidosis Acute kidney failure	Burns Diarrhoea
Sodium (Na^+)	135–145 mmol/L	Dehydration Reduced kidney function	Severe burns Overhydration

Table 9.4 Normal ranges for inorganic compounds in the plasma and causes of increase or decrease

Organic compound	Concentration	Increased	Decreased
Urea	2.5–8.5 mmol/L	High-protein diet Severe dehydration	Malnutrition Alcohol abuse
Uric acid Female Male	130–400 μmol/L 150–500 μmol/L	Glandular fever Lead poisoning	Coeliac disease Liver disease
Creatinine Female Male	50–110 μmol/L 55–145 μmol/L	Gout Diabetes	Muscle wasting Pregnancy
Bilirubin (total)	2–20 μmol/L	Hepatitis Cirrhosis	Not known

KEY POINTS

● There are many blood tests carried out to aid diagnosis and monitor treatment so it is important to be able to recognise results outside the normal range for the local laboratory.

● Specimens must be handled with care to avoid damaging the cells and must be sent to the laboratory as soon as possible.

● Make sure that the specimen and the form are labelled with the patient's details.

Glucose

Patients with diabetes need to keep their blood glucose as stable as possible in order to reduce the risk of complications. They have to balance their food intake, particularly starches and sugars, with their treatment. Patients are taught to monitor their blood glucose in capillary blood collected by piercing the *side* of a finger near the tip and dropping the blood onto a paper strip that has been impregnated with special chemicals. The strip is placed into a machine where it is read and the result displayed on a screen (**Figure 9.2**).

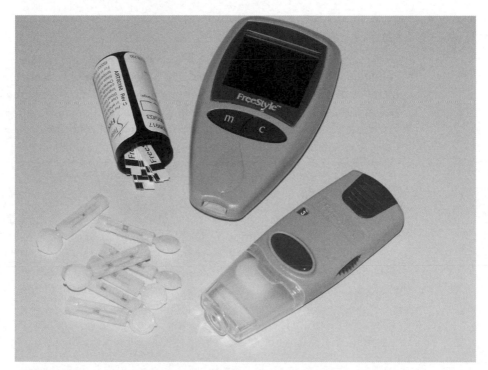

Figure 9.2 An example of a blood glucose monitor with reagent strips
Source: Phototake Inc./Alamy

There are many types of machines available, so you need to make sure that you understand the details of how they operate and have been trained to use them. The machines need regular calibration so make sure this has been done recently. Timings will differ as will the placement of the strip, so if you do not follow the instructions to the letter, the result will be wrong. This could be dangerous if the amount of insulin given depends on the result.

Blood glucose varies with the time of day and the time of and type of food taken in the last meal.

The normal range of fasting blood glucose is 3.5–5.5 mmol/L. If you measure it 2 hours after a meal it will rise but should be no more than 6 mmol/L. Patients with untreated diabetes may have a fasting level of 10 mmol/L or more and following food it may go up to 30 mmol/L or more.

A single recording does not reflect the control of glucose over time, which is an important consideration in preventing the complications associated with diabetes. The haemoglobin molecule becomes coated with glucose over time and can reflect on blood glucose levels over about a two month period. This type of haemoglobin is called HbA1c. Different laboratories have their own reference values for HbA1c, but most agree that the target value should be less than 6.5%.

Blood glucose may also rise in cases of extreme stress or trauma such as burns as the body tries to mobilise energy reserves. Patients may need a small dose of insulin to help return it to normal.

LOOK OUT

Make sure that the patient's fingers are clean and free from sugary contaminants. The patient's hands should be warm before collecting the blood so that you can obtain a good drop of blood. Stab the side of the finger because the tip of the finger is more sensitive and so it is more painful and if repeatedly stabbed can lead to loss of sensation. The ear lobe can also be used to collect capillary blood.

Metabolic rate

You have already seen in Chapter 8 how intake of food is vital to the well-being of patients. We use the energy from our food for driving our muscles, repairing tissues and for growth. The rate at which energy is used is called the metabolic rate.

Energy is released during the breakdown of nutrients, and oxygen is required for these reactions to occur with maximum efficiency. The amount of energy released when 1 litre of oxygen is used is approximately 20 kJ.

If we can measure the amount of oxygen used over a certain time, it is possible to estimate the amount of energy being released from the food. This is the metabolic rate.

Basal metabolic rate (BMR) is the measurement of metabolic rate under particular conditions and is used to see whether the rate is within the normal range. The subject has to be as quiet as possible so it is usually carried out before they get up. The subject must be lying down in a comfortably warm environment, not having had anything to eat or drink and as mentally relaxed as possible. Energy use is at its lowest point, basal, and can be compared with known rates for other people of a similar age, height, weight and gender.

Factors influencing metabolic rate

Gender – males have a higher metabolic rate than females.
   Metabolic rate can be increased above the basal rate by:

- Exercise – even a brisk walk can double the BMR and for a professional athlete by as much as 20 times.
- Hormones – thyroxine, adrenaline (epinephrine).
- Pregnancy.
- Digestion of food.
- Fever – a rise of 1°C increases metabolic rate by 10–15%.

It can be decreased by:

- Lack of exercise
- Depression.

BMR is measured in patients suspected of suffering from diseases affecting metabolic rate. In particular, oversecretion of thyroxine from the thyroid gland will increase metabolic rate making the patient have a rapid heart rate and feeling hot, whereas undersecretion will reduce metabolic rate slowing the heart and reducing body temperature. You can learn more about these conditions if you look at the BMR website.

APPLYING THE THEORY

Anaesthesia reduces metabolic rate, so particularly those patients undergoing long operations may suffer a drop in their temperature and shiver post-operatively in an attempt to generate heat with muscular activity. A low body temperature should be avoided as far as possible since it impacts on the maintaining of blood pressure.

   Elderly patients who move very little and very slowly have a reduced metabolic rate and may well feel cold even on a warm day. Feel the temperature of their legs if you don't believe me.

   The metabolic rate drops at night, and with it the body temperature. If you do night duty, you will find that at about 03:00 you will feel very cold and may even shiver. After a long stretch on nights, your body and temperature adjust.

9.2 URINALYSIS

Testing urine is a simple non-invasive way of assessing kidney function and detecting abnormalities that result from problems with other body systems.

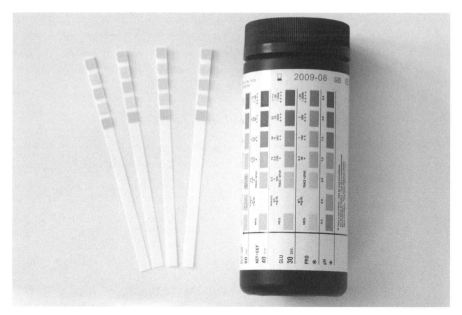

Figure 9.3 Reagent strips for urinalysis

Source: Mediscan

The specimen should be as clean as possible and tested soon after being collected. If the urine is to be sent to the laboratory for examination for possible infection, then special measures for collection should be carried out to ensure that it is
free from outside contamination. The most common method for ward testing is by
using chemically impregnated strips that are capable of monitoring between 2 and
11 different parameters.

The urine should be put into a clear container so that the test strip can be
immersed quickly. Excess urine should be tapped off, holding the strip horizontally
so that fluid from one pad does not contaminate the next. The strip can be read
from the colour chart on the side of the bottle (**Figure 9.3**) or by putting it into a
machine which has an optical reader which gives a printout of the results.

You must be supervised and tested by your mentor when using the equipment
and before carrying out testing on your own.

The timing of reading the strip from the chart is critical, so you must make sure
that you have a watch with a seconds hand available. The container should be
closed immediately after removing the strip to prevent moisture from the atmosphere degrading the chemicals in the strip.

The test strips can detect the following:

Specific gravity tells us about the amount of substances dissolved. This is
variable but is normally between 1005 and 1030. This is in comparison with pure
water which is 1000. In dehydration the specific gravity will increase and be low
in kidney failure.

pH is a reflection of the amount of acid or alkali being excreted by the kidneys
in order to maintain the pH of the blood at 7.4. Pure water has a pH of 7 which is

considered as the neutral point. A liquid with a pH of more than 7 is alkali, below 7 acid. The pH of urine is 5–6 but it will become more acidic during starvation and high-protein diet and more alkali with a vegetarian diet or in the presence of bacterial infection.

Blood in urine (**haematuria**) always needs to be investigated as it may be an early sign of bladder cancer, but there are other causes such as kidney stones.

Protein is found in urine in early kidney disease, but is commonly present in urinary tract infection. Proteinuria is a warning sign of pre-eclampsia, a potentially serious complication of pregnancy.

Glucose is not a normal finding in urine. Diabetes may be diagnosed first by finding glucose with a test strip but a more accurate test may be needed to estimate the actual amount of glucose in the circulation. Stress and severe trauma may also result in glycosuria – look again at the section on blood glucose.

Ketones are a waste product of fat metabolism. Normally the body uses glucose for energy but in fasting or a diet high in protein/low in carbohydrate fat is used instead. In poorly controlled diabetes, ketones are produced and can cause coma or death if left untreated.

Nitrites appear in the urine as a result of the breakdown of nitrates, which are a normal waste product. Nitrites appear as a result of bacteria in the urine, especially *Escherichia coli* which is a common cause of urinary tract infection.

The results of the test should be recorded in the patient's notes and any abnormalities reported to a senior member of staff.

9.3 BLOOD GASES

Respiratory disease is a common chronic problem that causes patients to be admitted to hospital. Monitoring the patient's respiration rate, peak expiratory flow rate and pulse oximetry are important observations that can be carried out on most wards, but sometimes it is important to use more detailed tests.

As you saw earlier in the chapter, the blood carries oxygen from the lungs to the tissues and removes waste carbon dioxide. If the lungs are not functioning properly then not enough oxygen can get to the tissues and the waste carbon dioxide builds up in the blood. Carbon dioxide makes the pH of the blood more acidic, which can be dangerous. Arterial blood gas measurement can help to monitor the severity of the disease and the response to treatment.

Atmospheric air is a mixture of gases, each taking up a different percentage of the total volume. This means that each contributes a different amount of pressure within the mix to form a total pressure of 103.1 kPa. The pressure of each gas is called the **partial pressure** of the gas (*P*) and is measured in kilopascals (kPa).

When air is breathed in, water vapour is added to the mix. When it reaches the air sacs in the lungs, the addition of carbon dioxide and the removal of oxygen into

Table 9.5 Percentage and partial pressure composition of atmospheric, alveolar and expired air

Gas	Atmospheric air		Alveolar air		Expired air	
	P(kPa)	%	P(kPa)	%	P(kPa)	%
O_2	21.2	20.9	13.3	13.1	15.6	15.4
N_2 (+noble gases)	79.6	78.6	76.4	75.3	75.6	74.6
CO_2	0.04	0.04	5.3	5.3	3.8	3.8
Water	0.5	0.5	6.3	6.2	6.3	6.2
Total	101.3	100	101.3	100	101.3	100

the blood change the proportions but the pressure remains at 101.3 kPa. The air that leaves the lungs contains a higher proportion of carbon dioxide and water vapour (**Table 9.5**).

Arterial blood gas estimation is carried out on a small sample of blood taken from an artery usually by a doctor and immediately analysed without allowing atmospheric air to contaminate the sample.

Normal values are

PCO_2 4.5–6.1 kPa PO_2 11.2–14.5 kPa

pH   7.35–7.45   bicarbonate (HCO_3^-)   22–28 mmol/L

A low pH gives the first indication of the presence of acidosis but does not tell you the cause. However, if the partial pressure of carbon dioxide (PCO_2) is raised then it is likely that there is a respiratory problem. The bicarbonate gives a base (alkali) balance to acidity to maintain the pH within normal levels. Bicarbonate levels below 22 mmol/L or above 26 mmol/L indicate a disturbance of metabolism.

LOOK OUT

If you know that an arterial blood sample is to be taken, you should be prepared to apply pressure to the sample site for at least 10 minutes in order to prevent bleeding and bruising. If a femoral artery has been used, this time may need to be longer because it is a large vessel under pressure. This procedure is more painful for the patient than the collection of venous blood so make sure that the patient is fully prepared.

Changes in atmospheric pressure

Atmospheric pressure varies, depending on how far from sea level it is measured, but the mix of gases stays the same. At sea level the pressure is 101.3 kPa in SI units but at the top of a 3000 m mountain it is about 70 kPa. This makes it less easy for oxygen to enter the circulation so the cells suffer **hypoxia** resulting in some climbers suffering from altitude sickness. People who live at high altitudes have more red cells per litre of blood than those who live at sea level, so that the oxygen-carrying power of the blood is increased.

If you dive, then the pressure is increased by 1 atmosphere for every 10 m depth so extra oxygen and nitrogen are pushed into the cells. Divers breathe from compressed air cylinders to equalise the pressure inside and outside the chest. If return to the surface is too rapid, the sudden release of pressure causes the gas to form bubbles in the tissues causing damage (it is very like the effect of undoing the top of a fizzy drink bottle). Decompression chambers are used, in cases where resurfacing has been too fast, to treat the condition called the bends. The pressure in the chamber is increased to 2 atmospheres, the same as at 10 m underwater, and then slowly returned to normal so that the gases return to solution.

RUNNING WORDS

albumen	glucose	partial pressure
anaesthesia	haematology	pH
anticoagulants	haematuria	plasma
arterial blood gas	haemoglobin	platelets
atmospheric pressure	homeostasis	protein
basal metabolic rate	hypoxia	prothrombin
differential count	interstitial fluid	reticulocytes
electrolytes	ketones	specific gravity
erythrocytes	nitrates	urinalysis
fibrinogen	organic	

Answers to the following questions can be found at the end of the book.

What did you learn?

(a) What is homeostasis? _____

(b) What are the solid parts of the blood? _____

(c) What percentage of the blood is taken up by these solids? _____

(d) Which proteins are involved in blood clotting? _____

(e) How many kilojoules are produced as a result of using a litre of oxygen in metabolic processes? _____

(f) Why would you suspect that *Escherichia coli* was present in a specimen of urine? _____

_____

(g) What percentage of atmospheric air is oxygen? _____

(h) What is wrong in the picture below?

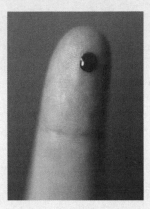

Source: Cristina Pedrazzini/
Science Photo Library

Web resources

http://www.patient.co.uk/showdoc/40025164/
Interesting website where you can find out more, not just about blood glucose monitoring but about management of diabetes, a disease that is on the increase.

http://www.fao.org/docrep/MEETING/004/M2845E/M2845E00.HTM
Learn more about oxygen uptake and BMR.

http://www.nursingtimes.net/ntclinical/2008/03/patient_assessment_part_6__
urinalysis.html
A comprehensive review of urinalysis.

http://www.webefit.com/Calculators/Calc_RestingMetaRate.html
A site for fun. You can calculate your own metabolic rate.

Suggested reading

Doherty L. and Lister S. (2008) *The Royal Marsden Manual of Clinical Nursing Procedures.* Chichester: Wiley-Blackwell.

Marieb E.N. and Hoehn K. (2007) *Human Anatomy and Physiology.* London: Pearson, Benjamin Cummings.

Chapter 10

Statistics and reading research articles

No ostriches here, please

In the first part of your programme you will not be expected to review research articles critically, but you will probably be asked to show an understanding of what you have read in your assignments. You should also be thinking about how what you read can be applied to improve practice.

When you have completed this chapter, you should be able to:

- State the difference between qualilative and quantitative research.

- Read a journal article in a systematic way.

- Understand how results of qualitative and quantitative data can be presented.

- Calculate the mean, median and mode.

- Appreciate the limitations of data presentation.

This chapter is a very gentle introduction to reading journal articles so that you can think about your clinical practice in relation to what you have read. You will certainly have much more detailed direction later on in your programme, so don't run away with the impression that this chapter is all you need to know – there are whole books on the subject.

Many of the articles you will read are not original research but small studies carried out by people who have some interest or expertise in the subject. Some will use statistics as a way of describing the information that has been collected about a particular topic or from designing and carrying out experiments. There are a few simple methods used to pull results together and so some of the commonest calculations and ways of presenting them will be discussed. **Statistical tests** help to decide the level of confidence that can be put on the results of an investigation, but don't panic – you won't have to do any or even read about them unless you want to look at the online resources.

Clinical practice needs to deliver the best possible care, so how do we know what makes care good? It is a requirement of professional bodies, such as the Nursing and Midwifery Council, that practice is evidence based.

What is evidence-based practice?

The way that care of individual patients is planned should be based on the current best evidence gained from research. The evidence should show that the treatment, care or procedures actually work rather than doing things in the way that they have always been done.

For example, it was thought that wounds healed best if you 'let the air get to them'. It is true that they will heal but it takes a long time, they get dry and crusty and the scab pulls and itches. You probably have had a wound like that and ended up picking the scab off! What happens then? It bleeds, so the process starts again. From research we now know that keeping the wound in a moist atmosphere (not wet) heals more quickly and is less painful.

That doesn't mean that the way you practise changes every time a piece of research is published because not all so-called research is good. There are a lot of steps in the process and one or more of these can be subject to errors of omission, inappropriate sampling, false conclusions – the list is endless. Clinical trials are specific types of research with strict criteria. What they are not is people trying out, say, a new dressing on a few patients to see how it performs.

You need to be able to read the latest research to both inform your practice and be able to make informed comment on articles for assignments. Later in your career you may have to undertake and write up a piece of research. (Yes, you!) This chapter should help you to begin to read and understand research.

Types of research

Research in healthcare falls into one of two camps: **quantitative** or **qualitative** research.

Table 10.1 Comparing quantitative and qualitative research

	Quantitative research	Qualitative research
Sample	Large numbers of specific data	Small numbers but detailed data
Data collection	Measurements of frequency, demographic data	Interviews, focus groups
Presentation of results	Statistics, graphs and tables	Themed comments

Quantitative research is chosen for things that can be measured or counted, e.g. the time taken for a surgical wound to heal using a particular dressing.

Qualitative research looks at the experiences of people, their feelings and their comments about a subject, e.g. how patients feel about being in a mixed-sex ward.

The way in which the two types of research differ can be seen in **Table 10.1**.

TIME TO TRY

Which type of research would be used to investigate the following subjects?

(a) The number of patients attending the A&E departments of 10 hospitals in England over a 6 month period.

(b) The experiences of patients attending the A&E department of a teaching hospital.

(c) The BMI of people with diabetes.

Answers: (a) quantitative (b) qualitative (c) quantitative.

10.1 READING A PAPER

A paper that arises as a result of the research process is published in journals of varying professional standing. Would you put more credibility on an investigation into a health-related topic if you read it in the *British Medical Journal* or *Heat* magazine?

There are a number of books and articles giving detailed advice about what to look for when reading a paper. This chapter gives a brief outline of the questions you need to keep in mind when doing your reading. The list is only a brief guide to begin to focus your reading so that later in your programme when you have to critically read articles you will have developed a systematic approach to the task.

Authors

● What are their academic or professional qualifications and expertise in the subject?

● Have they published other papers together, separately or with others?

Title

- Is the title clear and does tell it you what to expect in the paper?

Journal

- Is it a **peer-reviewed** journal, i.e. articles are critiqued by people of a similar professional background?
- Does the journal have a sponsorship that could **bias** the contributors? Is the article sponsored by a particular interest group or a company?

Abstract

- This is where you can decide whether or not the full article is what you need. The **abstract** should also contain key words to help you find related articles. This section is often available when you find articles online.

Introduction

- This section sets out the **hypothesis** or research question (which is not necessarily a question!), e.g. *This study aims to determine whether not shaving the skin pre-operatively is less likely to lead to post-operative infection than standard procedure.* It also should say why the author decided on this particular piece of research and why it is relevant to the area of professional practice. A comprehensive, up-to-date **literature review** should be included in the introduction, looking at previous research in the area and where the current research fits in.
- Is there any bias?
- Are all the sources of information listed in the reference section at the end?

Methods

Look at:

- How the authors choose the method of research?
- Did they do a pilot study to test out the **data collection tool**?
- What was the sampling method and was it appropriate for the type of study?
- Was the sampling size too small?
- How was the choice of subjects (people) made and was it appropriate for the study?
- Did all the subjects complete the study?
- Was **ethical permission** gained from the appropriate bodies, e.g. Trust Ethical Committee, University Ethical Committee?
- Was **consent** obtained from the subjects and how was confidentiality maintained?
- How was the data collected and was the tool (questionnaire, interview sheet, experiment) the right kind for collecting the information described?

- How was researcher bias removed?
- How reliable is the **data** and could it be **replicated** with similar results? (This is only relevant to quantitative data.)

This is the section to look at first if you need to determine if the work had been well prepared.

Results

- What the authors found.
- Are the results easy to read?
- Are the scales of the graphs appropriate?
- Is there any data excluded?

Discussion

- Does it reflect the title of the paper and the reason that the research was carried out?
- Are the statistics accurate and linked to the results?
- Do the authors discuss what they think the results mean?
- Does the discussion show bias or is some part of the results not discussed?
- Do the authors indicate any further research that could result from the study?

TIME TO TRY

Try it out before you have to do an assignment. Think of an area of practice that particularly interests you and find some papers to read.

Do they meet the above criteria? Do they give you any clear indication that you could improve practice? It might be helpful if you and some other students could read the same paper together and discuss your findings.

KEY POINTS

- Good clinical practice relies on understanding and applying best practice that is underpinned by research.
- Reading papers with a critical eye can help you to be aware of which information is reliable and could be used to improve the way you think about your care.

10.2 PRESENTATION OF DATA

One of the areas of a research paper that some people find more challenging is interpreting the results section because of the way in which the information is presented.

Qualitative data

There are a number of ways of presenting qualitative data: (i) **pie chart**, (ii) bar chart, (iii) proportional bar chart and (iv) **pictogram**.

A person's blood group is determined by the antigens on the outside of the erythrocytes (red cells). These give the blood group its name of A – has A antigen, B – has B antigen, AB – has both A and B antigens, but O has no antigens. In addition every blood group has or has not another antigen which gives the blood its rhesus type. Those individuals who have the rhesus factor are said to be rhesus positive and those without are rhesus negative. Approximately 15% of the population are rhesus negative.

What percentage of people are there in each ABO group? Put this data into a table (e.g. **Table 10.2**). It is much easier to see.

The data can be presented in different ways (**Figures 10.1(a)–(d)**). Which do you think shows the written information most clearly? Discuss this with your colleagues. You may find that some people understand one type of presentation more readily than another.

Table 10.2 Percentage of each of the ABO blood groups in the UK

Group	% of UK population	% Rh –ve
A	40	15%
B	11	15%
AB	4	15%
O	45	15%

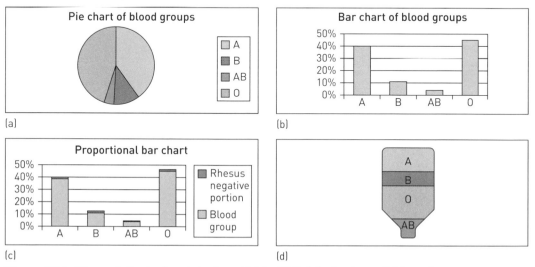

(a)

(b)

(c)

(d)

Figure 10.1 Ways of displaying data from Table 10.2: (a) pie chart; (b) bar chart; (c) proportional bar chart; and (d) pictogram – a 'blood bottle' divided to show the proportions of each blood group

Quantitative data

Quantitative data is not as easy to present as diagrams, especially if the data has a number of different characteristics. These are called **variables**.

Suppose you collected the heights of all the students in your tutorial group and wanted to display the results. Consider heights, in metres, of 12 students in the tutorial group. The variable in this case is the height of the student:

1.56   1.67   1.69   1.84   1.73   1.91   1.68   1.76   1.89   1.63   1.60   1.77

It is difficult to see any pattern in these results and you might criticise the size of the sample of students since it is quite small and generally quantitative research needs as many items as possible. The data we have here is the raw data, just as it was put down in the notebook at the time of measuring. Before it is presented for review or discussion of the results, the sample has to be regrouped.

Interval in metres*	Frequency
1.50–	0
1.55–	1
1.60–	2
1.65–	3
1.70–	1
1.75–	2
1.80–	1
1.85–	1
1.90–	1
1.95–	0

*The intervals represent up to 1.5 m but not including 1.55 m, 1.55 m up to but not including 1.60 m, and so on, otherwise there is confusion at the boundaries

The frequencies together form the frequency distribution, which in this case is 0, 1, 2, 3, 1, 2, 1, 1, 1, 0.

Now that the data is grouped, a diagram called a histogram can be drawn (**Figure 10.2**).

Bar charts and histograms may look similar but the histogram is used to illustrate quantitative data and the bar chart is used for qualitative data. In the histogram the boxes are next to each other but in a bar chart the bars are separate.

10.3 NORMAL DISTRIBUTION

You have looked at the heights of the tutorial group. How many adults do you know who are taller than 1.9 m or shorter than 1.5 m? Probably not as many as you know who are 1.65–1.85 m tall. We take it for granted that there is a range of heights in

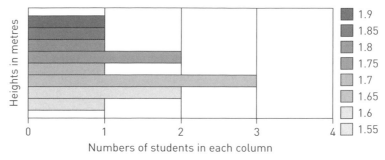

Figure 10.2 Histogram of heights of students in tutorial group

the population and that some people will be very short and some tall. We think of the range as normal – if we think about it at all.

The **normal distribution** of quantitative biological data has a few members at the extremes of the range and the bulk of the data equally distributed on either side of the midpoint. If the frequency data is plotted against the height for a sufficient number of people and the points joined together, the shape of the curve will be bell shaped. This is called a normal curve. **Figure 10.3** shows the normal distribution of IQ with the mean, 100, at the midpoint.

You will notice that the curve is inwards (concave) at each end and outwards (convex) at the top. The point at which the curve changes from concave to convex or convex to concave is called the point of inflection.

It is the shape of the curve that is important, not its relationship to the x-axis, since some parameters will not start at zero, e.g. height. You might have a few people with a height over 2 m and you might find some adults not much more than 1 m tall, but you won't have anyone of 0 m! In this case, the shape of the results is a

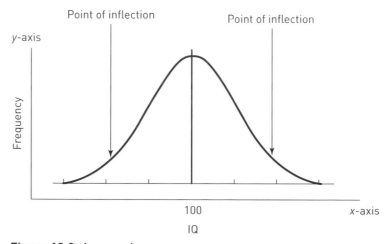

Figure 10.3 A normal curve

normal curve but it is shifted to the right of the graph. This is called a skewed normal curve.

APPLYING THE THEORY

When you take and record a patient's vital signs, you are comparing your findings with the normal range. This range has been calculated by taking the pulse rate of hundreds of people and plotting a frequency chart to form a bell-shaped normal curve.

Where is the middle?

In physiology normal is thought of as average and in statistics average is the **mean**. The mean, in a normal curve, is in the middle but it may not always be the centre of the range.

Find the mean of the following pulse rates:

62, 82, 74, 80, 60, 68, 76, 86, 68 beats per minute

First add all the data in the range and then divide the answer by the number of individual rates to find the mean. The sample of nine pulse rates in beats per minute is

$$62 + 82 + 74 + 80 + 60 + 68 + 76 + 86 + 68 = 656$$

Now divide 656 by 9 = 72.8. The mean of the data is 73 (correct to the nearest whole number). Is this the middle of the set?

The mean in this case is not one of the numbers in the results, nor is it the middle number. If we list the numbers in order, i.e. 60, 62, 68, 68, 74, 76, 80, 82, 86, it is called an **array**. The **median** is the middle value in an array, which in this case is 74. The median divides the array into two portions: half less than the median and half more than the median. Each half can be divided into two to form **quartiles**.

If there is an even number of values, then you take the two middle values in the array and the mean of the two is the median.

There is one more way of describing the average and that is the **mode**. The mode is the number that occurs most frequently in the data. In the sample of pulse rates above, the mode is 68.

In a normal distribution the mean, median and mode are the same.

TIME TO TRY

(a) Find the mean, median and mode of the following temperatures:

37°C, 35°C, 39°C, 36°C, 37°C, 38°C, 39°C, 37°C, 40°C

(i) mean = _____   (ii) median = _____   (iii) mode = _____

(b) What is the shape of a normal distribution curve? _____

(c) What are the common ways of displaying qualitative data? _____

_____

(d) What is the median of the following weights?

38 kg, 55 kg, 43 kg, 52 kg, 70 kg, 66 kg, 47 kg, 69 kg

Answers: (a) (i) 37.5°C (ii) 37.5°C (iii) 37°C (b) bell shaped (c) pie chart, bar chart, proportional bar chart, pictogram (d) 53.5 kg.

Beyond the 3Ms

Now you have got to grips with the mean, median and mode, you need to be able to recognise the abbreviations used in the presentation of data in research papers:

n is used for the number of results. What is *n* for the pulse rates in the example above?

Answer: *n* = 9.

x is used to represent a single observation of a variable *X*. The variable *X* that is being observed is the pulse rate and each rate is *x*, so when you see these in the results you will know what they represent.

The results of the pulse rates were added together and then divided by the number of results to find the mean. The Greek letter sigma Σ is used as shorthand for 'add together all the results'.

Σ*x* means add together all the observed values, which is the first stage in finding the mean. To find the mean, the added results are divided by the number of results, *n*.

$\frac{\Sigma x}{n}$ is the mean of all the values of *x* and is written, even more briefly, as $\bar{x}$ and called *x* bar.

TIME TO TRY

From the BMI recordings of 22, 34, 27, 24, 28, 30, what is the value of the following?

(a) *n* = _____   (b) $\bar{x}$ = _____

(c) Σ*x* = _____   (d) $\frac{\Sigma x}{n}$ = _____

Answers: (a) 6 (b) 27.5 (c) 165 (d) 27.5.

> **KEY POINTS**
>
> ● There are three ways of determining the middle of a range of data: mean, median and mode.
>
> ● They are not necessarily the same number and the mean and median may not equal any of the numbers in the range.
>
> ● The mean ($\bar{x}$) is found by identifying all the individual observations (x) of the variable (X), adding them together (Σ) and then dividing the sum by the number of observations (n).

Tricks of the trade

When you are reading graphs and tables, you should always be on the lookout for a misleading display of data. **Figure 10.4** shows weight loss following the 'lean and mean diet'. The first graph appears to show a creditable loss of weight but the same information in the second graph is not very impressive. Why? Graphs should always show the zero but on the y-axis graph (a) does not and this exaggerates the loss. That said, 0.7 kg in a week is considered a reasonable loss when dieting, but it won't be size 12 to 0 in a month!

Figure 10.5 is a graph of percentage hair growth that can be achieved using Hairgro. The graph starts at 10% but what is it 10% of? The final reading is 50% but

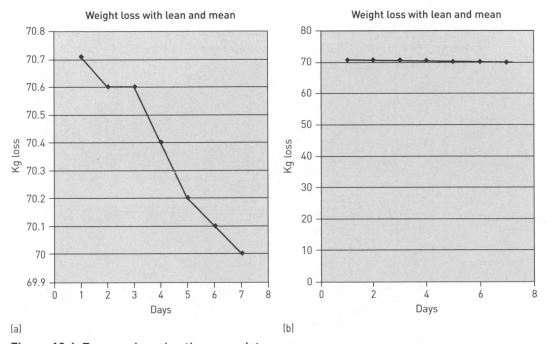

Figure 10.4 Two graphs using the same data

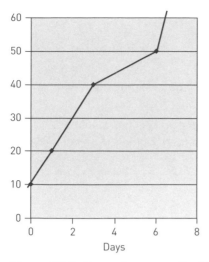

Figure 10.5 Percentage growth of hair using Hairgro

the line extends past the point and the angle at which it is set gives the impression of rapid growth. The extending of a graph in this way is called extrapolation.

Researchers often try to find a relationship between two variables such as the weight of a person and their cholesterol level. The relationship between two variables is known as **correlation**. When one variable is associated with an increase in another, it is said that there is a positive correlation. It does not mean that there is a cause and effect, though often such conclusions are made by the media. In **Figure 10.6** the points lie close to a straight line going through 0. Results like this from so few values would be suspect in real life. This type of relationship is called a positive correlation since the value of one variable increases as the other one does.

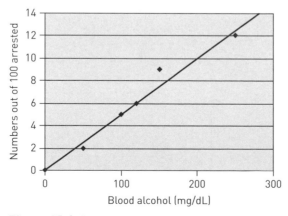

Figure 10.6 Numbers of arrests for alcohol-associated antisocial behaviour

In the case of this correlation, it might be concluded that the more alcohol is consumed, the more boys are arrested. Not necessarily so!

This type of correlation alerted Doll and Hill (1952) to the possible relationship between smoking and lung cancer which led to a long-term study of general practitioners and their smoking habits. It took several more years and statistical analyses of the data to convince a sceptical public that there was a cause and effect.

If the slope goes from a high value on the y-axis down towards the x-axis, then this is said to be a negative correlation. A decrease in one variable is associated with an increase in the other; for example, the soles on your shoes get thinner the further you walk.

Whether or not the relationship between the variables is correlated, the data is subjected to statistical tests. There are a number of tests that can be used but only one or two are suitable for the type of research undertaken and the results generated.

You will be glad to know that we are not going to do battle with those! However, there are some web resources if you are feeling brave.

As you go through your course, you will learn more about statistics on a need-to-know basis. There is no reason to be worried about it because, as you have seen in this chapter, you can learn the language one small step at a time and most calculations are only a variation of the ones that you managed in Chapters 1 and 2.

> ### RUNNING WORDS
>
> | | | |
> |---|---|---|
> | abstract | evidence-based practice | pictogram |
> | array | hypothesis | pie chart |
> | bias | literature review | qualitative |
> | consent | mean | quantitative |
> | correlation | median | quartiles |
> | data | mode | replicated |
> | data collection tool | normal distribution | statistical test |
> | ethical permission | peer reviewed | variable |

Answers to the following questions can be found at the end of the book.

What did you learn?

(a) What type of data would be classed as quantitative data?

_____

(b) In which section of a research paper would you expect to see the sampling discussed?

(c) What permissions are needed before research can be carried out? _____

_____

(d) Qualitative data is more suitably displayed in a bar chart or histogram? _____

(e) What is a point of inflection? _____

(f) How does the median divide the range? _____

(g) Put the following numbers into an array: 38, 20, 17, 43, 11, 29, 36, 30.

(h) Using the numbers in (g) above, what is

 (i) $n =$ _____ (ii) $\Sigma x =$ _____ (iii) $\bar{x} =$ _____?

Web resources

http://www.ms.uky.edu/~mai/java/stat/GaltonMachine.html
An animation of the formation of a normal curve – fun!

http://www.bbc.co.uk/schools/ks3bitesize/maths/handling_data/index.shtml
Look at the three sections on representing data and the two on averages for examples of pie charts, graphs and mean, mode and median.

http://www.bbc.co.uk/schools/gcsebitesize/maths/data/scatterdiagramsrev1.shtml
Learn more about positive and negative correlation.

http://www.graphpad.com/www/Book/Choose.htm
This is the place to go if you want to find out more about statistical tests.

http://www.bbc.co.uk/skillswise/numbers/handlingdata/graphs_and_charts/factsheet.shtml
This is a good place to start if you want more practice in reading and interpreting information from tables and charts. It helps you to read and extract information from some of the most challenging tables, e.g. bus and train timetables.

www.neighbourhood.statistics.gov.uk/
A good site for information about the area where you live or work. It puts statistics to use in a simple form.

Suggested reading

Cutcliffe J. and Ward M.F. (2007) *Critiquing Nursing Research*, 2nd edn. London: Quay Books.

Doll R. and Hill A.B. (1952) Study of aetiology of carcinoma of the lung. *British Medical Journal*, **2**: 1271–1286.

Doll R., Peto R., Boreham J. and Sutherland I. (2005) Mortality from cancer in relation to smoking: 50 years observations on British doctors. *British Journal of Cancer*, **34**: 426–429.

Greenhalgh T. (2006) *How to Read a Paper: The Basics of Evidence-Based Medicine*, 3rd edn. Oxford: Blackwell.

Laonë N. (2002) *Ogier's Reading Research*. London: Ballière Tindall.

Appendix A
Roman numerals and their Arabic equivalent

Roman numeral		Arabic numeral	Roman numeral		Arabic numeral
Upper case	Lower case		Upper case	Lower case	
I	i	1	XIV	xiv	14
II	ii	2	XV	xv	15
III	iii	3	XVI	xvi	16
IV	iv	4	XVII	xvii	17
V	v	5	XVIII	xviii	18
VI	vi	6	XIX	xix	19
VII	vii	7	XX	xx	20
VIII	viii	8	XXX	xxx	30
IX	ix	9	XL	xl	40
X	x	10	L	l	50
XI	xi	11	C	c	100
XII	xii	12	D	d	500
XIII	xiii	13	M	m	1000

In the Roman numeral system, the letters I, V and X are used in combinations to make the range of numbers up to 50.

The rules of combination are:

(a) When a letter is repeated it doubles its value and if repeated three times it triples its value:

$$X = 10 \qquad XX = 20 \qquad XXX = 30$$

(b) When the lower number comes before the higher number the values are subtracted:

$$V = 5 \qquad IV = 5 - 1 = 4$$

(c) If a lower number follows the higher number, they are added:

$$VI = 5 + 1 = 6$$

These rules apply to the larger numbers too:

$$XL = 50 - 10 = 40 \qquad MC = 1000 + 100 = 1100$$

The numbers can get cumbersome when they get bigger. Often at the end of a television programme the year in which the programme was made is written in Roman numerals. You can now look out for old films being recycled. If they do not start with MM (which equals 2000), then they were made in the last millennium. Which year was this?

$$MCMXCIX$$

Answer: 1999.

Appendix B
Multiples and divisions of SI units

Prefix	Abbreviation	Multiple or division	Factor
Yotta	Y	1 000 000 000 000 000 000 000 000	$= 10^{24}$
Zetta	Z	1 000 000 000 000 000 000 000	$= 10^{21}$
Exa	E	1 000 000 000 000 000 000	$= 10^{18}$
Peta	P	1 000 000 000 000 000	$= 10^{15}$
Tera	T	1 000 000 000 000	$= 10^{12}$
Giga	G	1 000 000 000	$= 10^{9}$
Mega	M	1 000 000	$= 10^{6}$
Kilo	k	1 000	$= 10^{3}$
Hecto	h	100	$= 10^{2}$
Deca	da	10	$= 10^{1}$
–	–	1	–
Deci	d	0.1	$= 10^{-1}$
Centi	c	0.01	$= 10^{-2}$
Milli	m	0.001	$= 10^{-3}$
Micro	μ	0.000 001	$= 10^{-6}$
Nano	n	0.000 000 001	$= 10^{-9}$
Pico	p	0.000 000 000 001	$= 10^{-12}$
Femto	f	0.000 000 000 000 001	$= 10^{-15}$
Atto	a	0.000 000 000 000 000 001	$= 10^{-18}$
Zepto	z	0.000 000 000 000 000 000 001	$= 10^{-21}$
Yocto	y	0.000 000 000 000 000 000 000 001	$= 10^{-24}$

Physical quantity	SI base unit	Symbol of SI unit
Length	Metre	m
Mass	Kilogram	kg
Volume	Cubic metre	m^3
Amount of substance	Mole	mol
Temperature	Kelvin	K

Equivalences of weight

1 kilogram (kg)	= 1000 grams	(g)
1 gram (g)	= 1000 milligrams	(mg)
1 milligram (mg)	= 1000 micrograms	(μg) – on prescriptions in full, microgram
1 microgram (μg)	= 1000 nanograms	(ng) – on prescriptions in full, nanogram

---

Equivalences of volume

1 litre (L)	= 1000 millilitres	(mL)
1 millilitre (mL)	= 1000 microlitres	(μL) – this should be written in full to prevent confusion with mL

Equivalences of length

1 metre (m)	= 1000 millimetres	(mm)
1 millimetre (mm)	= 1000 micrometres	(μm)
1 micrometre (μm)	= 1000 nanometres	(nm)

Centimetres (cm) are often used as a convenient fraction of a metre:

1 metre	= 100 centimetres
1 centimetre	= 10 mm

Multiplying by 1000

Move the decimal point to the right making the number bigger. As there are three zeros in 1000, the decimal point is moved three places:

73.0   730.0   7300.0   73 000.0

26.3   263.0   2630.0   26 300.0

Dividing by 1000

Move to the left making the number smaller:

73.0   7.3   0.73   0.073

26.3   2.63   0.263   0.0263

Appendix C
Important elements in the body

Element	Chemical symbol	Relative atomic mass	Percentage of body mass
Oxygen	O	16	65.0
Carbon	C	12	18.5
Hydrogen	H	1	9.5
Nitrogen	N	14	3.2
Calcium	Ca	40	1.5
Phosphorus	P	30.9	1.0
Sulphur	S	32	0.3
Sodium	Na	23	0.2
Chlorine	Cl	35.5	0.2
Magnesium	Mg	24	0.1
Iodine	I	127	0.1
Iron	Fe	55.9	0.1

Isotopes

Each element has its own relative atomic weight which is calculated by adding together the numbers of protons and neutrons in the centre of the atom.

For example, the atoms of carbon normally have six protons and six neutrons giving it a relative atomic mass of 12. There are some rogue atoms that have seven or eight neutrons, increasing the relative atomic mass of 13 or 14. Atoms of the same element that have different relatively atomic mass are called isotopes.

Some isotopes give out radioactive energy and are used for diagnosis or treatments. The iodine isotope I-131 is used to treat tumours of the thyroid gland.

Carbon is used as the standard for measuring the mole. A mole of carbon is the number of atoms in 12 g of the carbon-12 isotope.

Avogadro's constant

You are probably familiar with counting a certain number of items and giving them a name. We call a group of 24 hours a day, 7 days a week, or when you buy 12 Crispy Crème doughnuts, you have a dozen.

Think about two similar kinds of fruit, say oranges and satsumas. If you have a dozen of each, the oranges will take up a lot more space and weigh more than the satsumas, but you will have 12 of each.

Elements are made of atoms and the atomic mass in grams is called a mole. No matter what the relative atomic mass, a mole of a substance has a constant number of atoms, just like a dozen is always 12. (Yes, there is a baker's dozen!)

The number of atoms in 12 g of carbon (a mole) is 6.02×10^{23}. If this was written out in full it would be 602 000 000 000 000 000 000 000! This is known as Avogadro's constant. (You may also see it called Avogadro's number, which is the old name.)

Web resources

http://www.chem1.com/acad/webtext/intro/MOL.html
More examples of how to apply Avogadro's constant.

Appendix D
Reference values for adults

Haematology		
Erythrocyte sedimentation rate (ESR)	Female	3–15 mm/h
	Male	1–10 mm/h
Fibrinogen		1.5–4.0 g/L
Haemoglobin (Hb)	Female	120–160 g/L
	Male	130–175 g/L
Haematocrit (packed cell volume, PCV)	Female	37–48% 0.37–0.48 L/L
	Male	41–52% 0.41–0.52 L/L
Mean cell haemoglobin (MCH)		28–35 pg/cell
Mean cell volume		80–95 fL
Platelets (thrombocytes)		$150–350 \times 10^9/L$
Red blood cells (RBC) erythrocytes	Female	$3.9–5.5 \times 10^{12}/L$
	Male	$4.5–6.2 \times 10^{12}/L$
Reticulocytes (immature RBCs)		$25–85 \times 10^9/L$ 0.2–2% of RBC count
White cell (total)		$4.5–10.5 \times 10^9/L$
Differential white count	Neutrophils	45–75%
	Basophils	0–2%
	Eosinophils	0–6%
	Lymphocytes	20–45%
	Monocytes	2–10%

Biochemistry		
Albumen		34–46 gL
Bicarbonate		22–28 mmol/L
Bilirubin		3–16 μmol/L
Calcium		2.0–2.6 mmolL
PCO_2 (arterial)		4.5–6 kPa
Chloride		100–108 mmol/L
Cholesterol (total) fasting		Less than 5.2 mmol/L
Creatinine		55–145 μmol/L
Globulin		26–40 g/L
Glucose (fasting)		3.5–5.5 mmol/L
Glycosolated haemoglobin HbA1c		Less than 6.5%
Iron	Female	9.0–26 μmol/L
	Male	14–30 μmol/L
Magnesium		0.7–1.0 mmol/L
PO_2 (arterial)		11.2–14.5 kPa
Oxygen saturation		Greater than 98%
pH		7.35–7.45
Potassium		3.6–5.0 mmol/L
Protein (total)		60–80 g/L
Sodium		135–145 mmolL
Triglycerides (fasting)		0.6–1.8 mmol/L
Urea		2.5–6.5 mmol/L
Uric acid	Female	0.09–0.36 mmol/L
	Male	0.1–0.45 mmolL
Zinc		11–21 μmol/L

Note: There may be slight differences in these values in your practice area.

Appendix E
Abbreviations used in prescriptions

Abbreviation	Latin meaning	English translation	Note
a.c.	ante cibum	Before meals	
alt.die.	alterna die	Alternate days	
a.d.	auris dexter	Right ear	
a.s.	auris sinister	Left ear	
a.u.	auris utrae	Both ears	
b.d.	bis die	Twice daily	
b.i.d.	bis en die	Twice each day	
c.	cum	With	
cap.		Capsule	
c.c.	cum cibos	With food	Also means cubic centimetre
crem	cremor	Cream	
gtt.	guttae	Drops	
h.s.	hora somni	At bedtime	
inj.		Injection	
IMI		Intramuscular injection	
IU		International units	
IV		Intravenous	
man.	mane	Morning	
n.	nocte	Night	
neb.		To be nebulised	Made into droplets with air
oc.	oculentum	Eye ointment	
O.D.	omni dei	Every day	See o.d. below
o.d.	oculus dexter	Right eye	See O.D. above
o.m.	omni mane	Every morning	
o.n.	omni nocte	Every night	
o.s.	oculus sinister	Left eye	
p.c.	post cibum	After meals	
p.o.	per os	By mouth	

Abbreviation	Latin meaning	English translation	Note
p.r.	per rectum	Rectally	
p.r.n.	per re nata	As needed	Frequency and maximum dose should be specified
pulv.	pulivis	Powder	
p.v.	per vaginum	Vaginally	
q.	quaque	Every	
q.d.	quaque die	Every day	
q.d.s.	quarter die sumendus	Four times a day	
q.h.	quaque hora	Every hour	q3h–every 3 hours, q4h . . .
q.i.d.	quarter in die	Four times a day	
S.C.		Subcutaneous	
S.L.		Sublingually – under the tongue	
s.o.s.	sit opus sit	If needed	Frequency and maximum dose should be specified
stat.	slalum	At once	
supp.	suppoaitorium	Suppositories	
tab.		Tablet	
TDD		Total daily dose	
t.d.s.	ter die sumendus	Three times a day	
t.i.d.	ter in die	Three times a day	
top.		Topically	On the skin's surface
ung.	ungmentum	Ointment	

Note: These abbreviations are being used less frequently but you will still see them on prescriptions.

Appendix F
An example of a medicine chart

City Hospital
Drug Prescription and
Administration Record

Surname   GREENWAY
First name   Amanda
Hosp. no.   C123456
Date of birth   12/12/50

Drug Idiosyncrasy				Ward *Albert*		Sheet no. 1
Drug	Type of reaction	Source of information	Signature	Consultant *Mr Goodwin*		
PENICILLIN	*Rash*	*Patient*	*A Doctor*	House Officer Dr Munday		
				Date of admission	Day *01*	Month *01*	Year *2009*
				Weight *68kg*	Height *1.55m*	Surface area *1.6m²*
				BMI *28*		
				Pregnancy *n/a*		Breast feeding *n/a*
Special diet *none*				TTOs to Pharmacy		For delivery by
				Date		Date

(Surface area shown as $1.6\,m^2$)

Once only drugs and premedications

Date	Time	Drug	Dose	Route	Prescriber's signature	Given by	Time given	Pharm.
01.01.09	15:00	DIAMORPHINE	20mg	IV	JMunday	jlm	15:00	

Medical gases

Gas	Flow rate	% Mask or nasal cannulae	Additional instructions	Signature
Oxygen	6L/min	cannulae	Humidified	JMunday

As required prescriptions

Drug (approved name) PARACETAMOL			Date 01/01/09		02/01/0							
Dose 1g	Route orally	Frequency 4-6 hourly	Pharm.	Time	20:00							
Additional instructions Not more than 4g in any 24 hours			Dose and route administered		1g 0							
Prescriber's signature JMunday	Start date 01/01/09		Finish date 05/01/09	Given by								
Drug (approved name)			Date									
Dose	Route	Frequency	Pharm.	Time								
Additional instructions			Dose and route administered									
Prescriber's signature	Start date		Finish date	Given by								
Drug (approved name)			Date									
Dose	Route	Frequency	Pharm.	Time								
Additional instructions			Dose and route administered									
Prescriber's signature	Start date		Finish date	Given by								
Drug (approved name)			Date									
Dose	Route	Frequency	Pharm.	Time								
Additional instructions			Dose and route administered									
Prescriber's signature	Start date		Finish date	Given by								
Drug (approved name)			Date									
Dose	Route	Frequency	Pharm.	Time								
Additional instructions			Dose and route administered									
Prescriber's signature	Start date		Finish date	Given by								
Drug (approved name)			Date									
Dose	Route	Frequency	Pharm.	Time								
Additional instructions			Dose and route administered									
Prescriber's signature	Start date		Finish date	Given by								

NOTES TO PRESCRIBERS FOR THE SAFETY OF THE PATIENT:

1. The prescription must be **CLEARLY** written in **CAPITAL LETTERS** using the **APPROVED NAME** of the drug.
2. If a prescription is cancelled it must be **CROSSED OUT, DATED** and **INITIALLED.**
3. Where prescriptions need to be changed, they should be **CANCELLED** and **REWRITTEN.**
4. Only **ONE** prescription sheet should be in use for each patient. If a new chart is required, then **CROSS OUT EACH PAGE** of the old chart and give a **sequential number** to the new prescription sheet.

Regular prescriptions

Date and month				01/01/09											
Tick times or enter variation ⟶															
Drug (approved name) *CEFRADINE*			6 ✓												
			8												
Dose *500 mg*	Route *oral*	Pharmacy	12 ✓	*JM*											
Prescriber's signature *JMunday*			14												
			18 ✓	*JM*											
Start date *01/01/09 12:00*	Finish date *06/01/09* *06:00*		22 24 ✓	*JM*											
Drug (approved name)			6												
			8												
Dose	Route	Pharmacy	12												
Prescriber's signature			14												
			18												
Start date	Finish date		22												
Drug (approved name)			6												
			8												
Dose	Route	Pharmacy	12												
Prescriber's signature			14												
			18												
Start date	Finish date		22												

Key for medication not given – to be entered in red ink. A – absent from ward, N – nil by mouth, O – not required, P – patient unable, R – refused, U – drug unavailable. Nurse in charge must be notified of omissions.

Infusion therapy

Date	Intravenous fluid	Volume	Duration	Additives and dose	Prescriber's signature	Batch number	Nurse's signature	Time started	Time completed	Pharmacist
01/01/09	Normal Saline	1 litre	4 hours	none	JMunday	C098/45	AMason	07.30	11.40	
01/01/09	5% Dextrose	1 litre	6 hours	none	JMunday	s0774/69	H Shepherd	11.45		

Appendix G
Peak expiratory flow rate

PEAK EXPIRATORY FLOW RATE - NORMAL VALUES
For use with EU/ISO 23747 scale PEF meters only

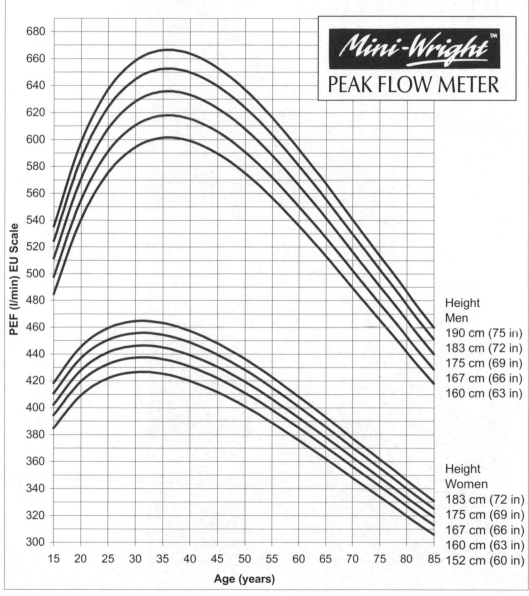

Source: Adapted by Clement Clarke for use with EN13826/EU scale peak flow meters from Nunn A.J. and Gregg I. (1989)
Br Med J, **298**: 1068–70.
Clement Clarke International Ltd

Appendix H
Body mass index and Malnutrition Universal Screening Tool (MUST)

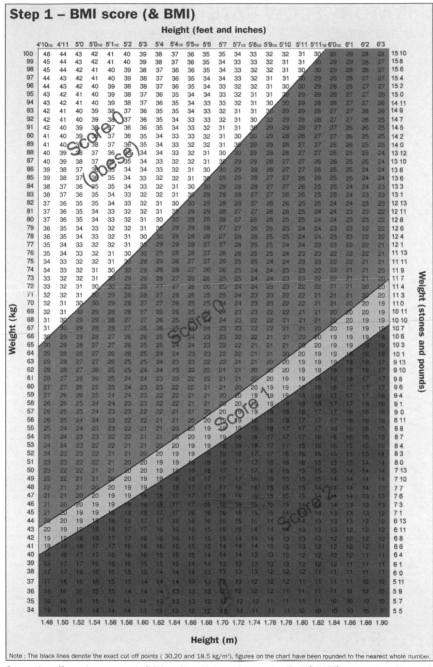

Source: http://www.bapen.org.uk. 'Malnutrition Universal Screening Tool' (MUST) is reproduced here with the kind permission of BAPEN (British Association for Parenteral and Enteral Nutrition)

Appendix I
Nomogram for calculating body surface area

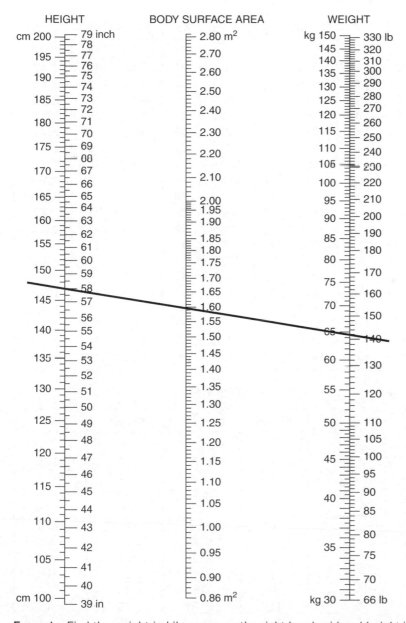

Example: Find the weight in kilograms on the right hand grid and height in centimetres on the left hand grid. Join the two with a straight line and read the body surface area from the centre column. Weight = 64.5 kg; Height = 147 cm; Body Surface Area = 1.59 m².

Appendix J
Weight conversion tables

Conversion of kilograms to pounds

Kg	Pounds	Kg	Pounds	Kg	Pounds	Kg	Pounds	Kg	Pounds	Kg	Pounds
1	2.2	21	46.2	41	90.2	61	134.2	81	178.2	101	222.2
2	4.4	22	48.4	42	92.4	62	136.4	82	180.4	102	224.4
3	6.6	23	50.6	43	94.6	63	138.6	83	182.6	103	226.6
4	8.8	24	52.8	44	96.8	64	140.8	84	184.8	104	228.8
5	11.0	25	55.0	45	99.0	65	143.0	85	187.0	105	231.0
6	13.2	26	57.2	46	101.2	66	145.2	86	189.2	106	233.2
7	15.4	27	59.4	47	103.4	67	147.4	87	191.4	107	235.4
8	17.6	28	61.6	48	105.6	68	149.6	88	193.3	108	237.6
9	19.8	29	63.8	49	107.8	69	151.8	89	195.8	109	239.8
10	22.0	30	66.0	50	110.0	70	154.0	90	198.0	110	242.0
11	24.2	31	68.2	51	112.2	71	156.2	91	200.2	111	244.2
12	26.4	32	70.4	52	114.4	72	158.4	92	202.4	112	246.4
13	28.6	33	72.6	53	116.6	73	160.6	93	204.6	113	248.6
14	30.8	34	74.8	54	118.8	74	162.8	94	206.8	114	250.8
15	33.0	35	77.0	55	121.0	75	165.0	95	209.0	115	253.0
16	35.2	36	79.2	56	123.2	76	167.2	96	211.2	116	255.2
17	37.4	37	81.4	57	125.4	77	169.4	97	213.4	117	257.4
18	39.6	38	83.6	58	127.6	78	171.6	98	215.6	118	259.6
19	41.8	39	85.8	59	129.8	79	173.8	99	217.8	119	261.8
20	44.0	40	88.0	60	132.0	80	176.0	100	220.0	120	264.0

Pounds to kilograms

Pounds	Kg
1	0.45
2	0.9
3	1.35
4	1.8
5	2.25
6	2.7
7	3.15
8	3.6
9	4.05
10	4.5
11	4.95
12	5.4
13	5.85
14 (1 stone)	6.35

Stones to kilograms

Stones	Kg	Stones	Kg
1	6.35	15	95.25
2	12.7	16	101.6
3	19.1	17	107.95
4	25.4	18	114.3
5	31.75	19	120.65
6	38.1	20	127.0
7	44.45	21	133.35
8	50.8	22	139.7
9	57.15	23	146.0
10	63.5	24	152.4
11	69.89	25	158.75
12	76.2	26	165.1
13	82.55	27	171.46
14	88.9	28	177.8

Appendix K
Summary of methods for drug calculations

If the prescribed drug and the dose on the medicine container are in different units, change the larger one to smaller units to avoid decimal points.

(a) Tablets/capsules

$$\frac{\text{amount of drug prescribed}}{\text{amount of drug in each tablet/capsule}} = \text{number of tablets or capsules}$$

A patient is prescribed aspirin 600 mg. The tablets are 300 mg each. How many tablets will you give?

$$\frac{600\ \text{mg}}{300\ \text{mg}} = 2\ \text{tablets}$$

(b) Liquid medicines

$$\frac{\text{amount of drug prescribed}}{\text{amount of drug in each unit}} \times \frac{\text{volume the drug is in (e.g. 1 mL, 5 mL)}}{1}$$

$$= \text{volume of drug required}$$

A patient is prescribed amoxicillin 250 mg. The bottle label reads 125 mg in 5 mL. How much will you give?

$$\frac{250\ \text{mg}}{125\ \text{mg}} \times \frac{5\ \text{mL}}{1} = 10\ \text{mL}$$

(c) Drugs prescribed according to **body surface area**

$$\text{surface area in } m^2 \times \text{dose per } m^2 = \text{dose in grams or milligrams}$$

Calculate the dose of a drug to be given to a patient with a surface area of 1.55 m^2 and prescribed 250 mg/m^2:

$$1.55 \times 250\ \text{mg} = 387.5\ \text{mg}$$

Now work out the amount to be given as in (a) or (b) above, as appropriate.

(d) Drugs prescribed according to **body weight**

body weight in kg (or g if an infant) × dose per kg (or g)

Calculate the dose of the drug to be given if a patient weighing 73 kg is prescribed a dose of 5 mg/kg:

$$73 \times 5 \text{ mg} = 365 \text{ mg}$$

Drugs prescribed using surface area or weight may be given as the calculated dose a number of times per day, or the dose calculated may be for the *whole* day and needs to be split into *several* doses over the course of the day – **CHECK**.

Calculating the rate of flow for intravenous fluids

Intravenous giving sets are calibrated to deliver 20 drops per millilitre of fluid and are used for clear fluids.

You need to know, from the prescription, the volume of fluid to be given (in millilitres) and the time over which it has to be given (in minutes):

$$\frac{\text{number of millilitres to be given} \times \text{drops per mL of the giving set}}{\text{number of minutes}} = \text{drops per minute}$$

A patient is prescribed 1 L 5% glucose to be given over 4 hours. How many drops per minute should be given?

$$\frac{1000 \times 20 \text{ drops}}{4 \times 60 \text{ minutes}} = 83.3 = 83 \text{ drops per minute}$$

Micro-drop delivery sets are calibrated to deliver 60 drops per millilitre of fluid and are used for paediatric fluid administration and drug delivery in adults.

You need to know, from the prescription, the volume of fluid to be given (in millilitres) and the time over which it has to be given (in minutes):

$$\frac{\text{number of millilitres to be given} \times \text{drops per mL of the giving set}}{\text{number of minutes}} = \text{drops per minute}$$

A patient is prescribed 100 mL of fluid to be given over 2 hours. How many drops per minute should be given?

$$\frac{100 \times 60 \text{ drops}}{2 \times 60 \text{ minutes}} = 50 \text{ drops per minute}$$

Blood administration sets have a filter chamber and are calibrated to deliver 15 drops per mL.

You need to know, from the prescription, the volume of fluid to be given (in millilitres) and the time over which it has to be given (in minutes):

$$\frac{\text{number of millilitres to be given} \times \text{drops per mL of the giving set}}{\text{number of minutes}} = \text{drops per minute}$$

A patient is prescribed 450 mL blood which is to be given over 4 hours. How many drops per minute should be given?

$$\frac{450 \times 15 \text{ drops}}{4 \times 60 \text{ minutes}} = 28.125 = 28 \text{ drops per minute}$$

Volumetric pumps deliver intravenous fluid in millilitres per hour.

You need to know, from the prescription, the volume of fluid to be given (in millilitres) and the time over which it has to be given (in hours):

number of millilitres to be given $\div$ number of hours = millilitres per hour

A patient is prescribed 1 L of 0.9% saline over 4 hours. At how many millilitres per hour should the machine be set?

$$1000 \div 4 = 250 \text{ mL per hour}$$

Glossary

% volume in volume (% v/v) A volume of concentrate (in mL) that has to be mixed with water to make 100 mL.

% weight in volume (% w/v) The amount of solid (in g) that is mixed with water to make 100 mL solution.

% weight in weight (% w/w) The amount of solid (in g) that must be mixed with another solid to make 100 g.

1 in 4 A solution in which there is one part of concentrate mixed with three parts of water to make a total of four parts.

1 to 4 or 1:4 A solution in which one part of concentrate is mixed with four parts of water to make a total of five parts.

abstract A section of a research paper containing key words and a synopsis of the study undertaken.

addition The mathematical process of finding the total of two or more numbers. Other words that have a similar meaning are sum of, plus, altogether, increase by.

adrenaline (epinephrine) A naturally occurring hormone that stimulates the autonomic nervous system in stressful situations. It is also used as a treatment to constrict blood vessels to reduce bleeding.

albumen A major blood protein that is important in maintaining fluid in the circulation.

ampoule A type of glass or plastic container for liquid drugs or sterile water.

anaesthesia Drug-induced loss of consciousness to prevent sensation of pain. Sometimes used incorrectly to describe local analgesia.

anticoagulant A drug used to increase the time that blood takes to coagulate (clot).

array A list of numbers in numerical order.

arterial blood gas The level of oxygen and carbon dioxide in the arterial circulation.

atmospheric pressure The amount of downward pressure exerted by the combined pressure of gases in the atmosphere.

atom The smallest part of an element that shows the characteristics of the element. Atoms are composed of protons, neutrons and electrons.

axilla The correct name for the armpit.

basal metabolic rate The speed at which the body uses energy at complete rest.

base 10 The number system based on groups of tens.

beam balance Weighing scales that involve moving weights along bars until they are balanced against the mass on the scale pan or platform.

bias The inclination towards or against a particular result by flaws in the design or sampling analysis of any part of the research process.

biphasic A mixture of short- and long-acting insulin.

blood glucose The way in which carbohydrates are carried in the blood. It is maintained at a steady level by insulin.

blood pressure The force exerted by the circulating blood on the walls of the arteries.

BMI Body Mass Index is calculated by dividing an individual's body weight (in kg) by their height in metres squared (m^2). Normal range is 20–25.

BODMAS A mnemonic for the order in which to carry out a calculation containing different types of mathematical process: Brackets, Other operations, Division, Multiplication, Addition, Subtraction.

body surface area The area of skin covering the body. It varies with height and weight.

borrowing A process that you may need to use when subtracting, if the number on the bottom is larger than that on the top.

bradycardia A heart rate below 60 beats per minute.

burette A type of intravenous fluid giving set used to deliver small volumes of fluid.

calibration A method of ensuring that equipment is functioning correctly by comparing and adjusting it with a known standard.

carrying over When the sum of a column of figures is greater than 10, the 'extra' is added to the next column.

chlorhexadine An antiseptic which may need to be diluted before use.

common denominator A number that can be used to make fractions that have different denominators equal fractions with the same number or common denominator, e.g. $2/3 + 1/4$ can have a common denominator of 12 making them into equivalent fractions of $8/12$ and $3/12$.

compound drug A medicine that contains two or more drugs.

consent An important feature in care delivery and research, whereby permission must be sought from the patient before an intervention or participation in the research process.

contusion The correct name for bruising.

correct to two decimal places Making a long decimal fraction manageable and acceptably accurate by correcting the number to two decimal places, e.g. 1.785 correct to two decimal places is 1.79.

correlation The relationship between two variables, e.g. smoking and the development of lung cancer.

counting on A method of adding, by starting with the larger number and counting on the number of the second.

cross-infection The passing of infection from one infected site to a vulnerable individual.

data Facts or quantities that are collected and analysed.

data collection tool Questionnaires, tables and other kinds of recording methods to gather information in carrying out research.

dead space The volume of air that is moved in and out during respiration without reaching the lungs.

decimal fraction A part of a number that is written after the decimal point, e.g. £3.50.

denominator The number that is below the line in a vulgar fraction, e.g. in $\frac{1}{5}$, 5 is the denominator.

diastolic pressure The lower reading of the blood pressure recording, produced when the ventricles of the heart are not contracting.

differential count The number of each type of white blood cell in a sample of blood.

displacement value The volume in a solution that is taken up by the substance that is dissolved and must be taken into account when preparing drugs for injection.

diuretic A drug used to increase the output of urine.

dividend The number that is to be divided in a division. In the sum 12 divided by 6, **12** is the dividend.

division Sharing. For example, if you have 12 apples and six people to share them among equally then you divide the number of apples by the number of people: 12 divided by 6 gives the answer 2.

divisor The number that does the dividing in a division. In the sum 12 divided by 6, **6** is the divisor.

drops per minute The rate that needs to be calculated in order to deliver a prescribed volume of intravenous fluid over a given amount of time.

drug strength The amount of drug contained in a particular volume/tablet/capsule.

dyspnoea Difficulty in breathing.

electrolytes Chemicals such as salts, acids and bases that dissociate (break up) in water and are able to carry an electric charge.

element A member of a limited number of substances from which all other substances are made, e.g. oxygen, hydrogen, carbon.

energy The amount of heat that is contained in food that can be used to drive body processes.

enteral The intestinal route for drug administration.

enteric coated Drugs coated to prevent their being destroyed by the acid in the stomach.

epistaxis The correct term for a nose bleed.

equivalent fractions Fractions that, if simplified, result in the same fraction, e.g. 2/4, 3/6, 5/10 can all be simplified to 1/2.

erythrocyte Red blood corpuscles (cells).

ethical permission The permission that must be sought from the appropriate bodies before research can be carried out.

evidence-based practice The conscientious, explicit and careful use of current best information to underpin decisions about the care of individual patients.

expiration The process of breathing out.

exponent Shorthand for multiplication, e.g. $5 \times 5 = 5^2$, $5 \times 5 \times 5 = 5^3$. The 'exponent' stands for however many times the number is being multiplied. The number that is being multiplied is called the 'base'.

FEV$_1$ Forced Expiratory Volume in 1 second gives an indication of the condition of a patient's airways.

fibrinogen A blood protein that takes part in blood clotting.

fluid balance The difference between the amount of fluid taken into the body and that excreted.

fluid overload Excess fluid retained in the body.

forced vital capacity (FVC) The volume of air that is expelled from the lungs with maximum effort and speed after a full inspiration. The volume and rate of expiration is reduced in chronic respiratory disease.

formula A shorthand method of describing the structure of a chemical, e.g. water H_2O, sodium chloride (salt) NaCl.

formulation The method of presenting drugs, e.g. tablets, capsules, liquid medicine.

generics Drugs which are produced by several manufacturers. Also known as non-proprietary name.

glucose The form in which carbohydrate from the diet is carried in the blood. Its level is controlled by the production of insulin.

gravity The force that attracts a body towards the centre of the Earth.

haematology The study of the solid elements in blood.

haematuria The presence of blood in urine.

haemoglobin A compound that contains iron, found in erythrocytes. It carries oxygen from the lungs to the tissues.

heparin A naturally occurring anticoagulant which is also given as treatment for thrombosis.

homeostasis The balancing forces in the body that keep parameters such as temperature, blood glucose and heart rate within a range that is considered normal.

hypertension A blood pressure that is higher than normal.

hypotension A blood pressure that is lower than normal.

hypothesis The formal statement of expected outcomes of the research question or proposal.

hypoxia The condition in which there is a reduction in the amount of oxygen available to the tissues.

improper fraction A fraction where the figure on the top line (numerator) is larger than the number on the bottom (denominator), e.g. $\frac{24}{6}$.

indices Singular, index. This is another way of describing an exponent.

insensible loss The amount of fluid lost from the body without the individual being aware, e.g. sweat, respiration.

insulin A naturally occurring hormone that controls blood glucose. It is also used to manage diabetes.

insulin syringe A special syringe graduated in units rather than millilitres, used only for insulin administration.

interstitial fluid The part of the body fluid that surrounds the individual cells of the tissues.

intravenous (IV) fluids Fluids that are given directly into a vein.

inverted Turning upside down, e.g. when dividing fractions, the dividing fraction is inverted before multiplying.

ketones Waste product of fat metabolism.

lidocaine A drug that produces local analgesia.

literature review An important prelude to carrying out research where previous related research is identified and reviewed in order to clarify where the current proposal fits in.

low molecular weight heparin (LMWH) A type of anticoagulant with smaller particles than standard heparin.

Luer-lock A type of locking connection between a syringe or other fluid administration device.

mean The result obtained by adding together all the values of the data and then dividing the total by the number of values (average).

median The result of putting the individual data in order from the smallest to the largest and selecting the value that is in the middle.

meniscus The curve in the surface of a liquid in a container, produced by the action of surface tension. It has two lines. In order to measure accurately, the lower line of the curve is read against the scale.

micro-drop administration set An intravenous fluid administration set that is calibrated to release 60 drops per millilitre of fluid.

milliequivalent Used in the United States as a measurement instead of the milllimole. Note that they are not equivalent in all cases.

mixed number A number that contains a whole number and a fraction, e.g. $3\frac{2}{3}$.

mmHg Millimetres of mercury. The unit used to measure blood pressure.

mode This is the value that occurs most frequently in a set of data.

mole (mol) A mole of an element or compound is equal to its atomic or molecular weight in grams.

multiplication Groups of, product, or times, all mean multiply. Multiplication is a quick method of addition: 3×4 means three lots of four or four lots of three. You could write this as $4 + 4 + 4$ or $3 + 3 + 3 + 3$; the answer is the same, 12.

near number Using a number that is easy to calculate in your head and close to the number being used so that you can check that your answer is sensible, especially when using a calculator, e.g. $152 + 127$ could be seen as $150 + 130 = 280$. The actual answer is 279.

negative number A number that is less than zero, such as in a temperature below zero. In the winter the temperature is often $-5°C$.

nitrates Chemicals found in urine which may indicate the presence of infection.

nomogram A chart that makes complex calculations simple, e.g. finding body surface area from height and weight.

non-proprietary name The common name for a drug, also known as the generic name.

normal distribution The way in which data is distributed evenly either side of the midpoint to form a bell-shaped curve.

number bond The way in which a set of numbers can be added together to form the same total, e.g. $1 + 9 = 10$, $4 + 6 = 10$, $8 + 2 = 10$ or $15 + 5 = 20$, $12 + 8 = 20$.

numeral Another name for a single number.

numerator The number on the top line of a fraction, e.g. in $\frac{3}{8}$, 3 is the numerator.

oral syringe A syringe designed so that it cannot be fitted with a needle and used to give accurate doses of liquid medicines.

organic Substances that are made up of compounds containing carbon.

oxygen saturation The percentage of oxygen carried by the red blood cells. This is normally 98% or more.

parenteral The way in which drugs are given via routes other than orally, e.g. subcutaneous, intramuscular.

partial pressure The fraction of pressure contributed to the whole by one component.

partitioning Breaking up numbers to a manageable size and subtracting them in turn.

patient-controlled analgesia (PCA) A method of pain relief whereby a patient is able to control delivery of the drug.

peer review The process of experts in a particular field reviewing the quality of work of others submitted for publication.

per cent An amount in or for every hundred.

percentage The rate per hundred or a share of the whole.

pH The measure of relative acidity or alkalinity of a solution.

pictogram A representation of data in the form of a picture.

pie chart Data presented in the form of a circle divided into representative portions of the whole, like slices of a pie.

place holder A zero used when there is no other to ensure that other numbers maintain their position, e.g. 10 (see place value).

place value It tells us what 'a number is worth', depending on where in a line of numbers it is written, e.g. 5 has a different value if it is in the number 157 or 568. It has moved from being 5 units, to 50 to 500.

plasma The fluid component of the blood, containing dissolved salts and other soluble substances.

platelets Small cell fragments in the blood that are involved in clotting (also known as thrombocytes).

positive number A number that is greater than zero.

prefix A group of letters placed before a word that indicates the size of the unit being used, e.g. milli, meaning one-thousandth of the unit, or centi, meaning one-hundredth, as in millilitre – one-thousandth of a litre.

prophylaxis Action taken to prevent a disease or condition.

proprietary name The name of a drug given by the manufacturer which first produced the medicine, e.g. Panadol, which is now made by several companies under its generic or non-proprietary name of paracetamol.

protein The only nutrient that contains nitrogen and is used for tissue repair and growth. It is broken down during digestion into its component parts, called amino acids.

prothrombin A blood protein that is involved in blood clotting.

pulse oximeter A device that is placed on a finger to measure the oxygen saturation of the haemoglobin.

qualitative A type of research where the information is gathered in depth from individuals.

quantitative A type of research where the information is gathered, ideally from a large number of individuals, and involves measurements.

quartiles The median splits the data into two equal parts. Each of these parts can be split into two, each called a quartile.

quotient The result or answer when one number is divided by another, e.g. the quotient of 10 divided by 5 is 2.

radial artery The artery that lies over the radius (the bone on the outside of the forearm when the palm faces upwards) and commonly used to calculate the pulse rate.

ratio The relationship between two numbers showing the number of times that one value is contained in the other.

recombinant DNA A method of using genetic material to produce drugs, e.g. insulin.

relative atomic mass The ratio of the average mass of one atom of an element to one-twelfth of the mass of an atom of carbon-12, e.g. oxygen 16, hydrogen 1.

relative formula mass The total of the relative atomic masses of the components in a compound, e.g. for water, H_2O (two lots of hydrogen 2 plus oxygen 16), the relative formula mass is 18.

replicated The ability to reproduce the results of an experiment by another researcher.

reticulocytes Immature red blood cells.

scientific calculator A hand-held calculator that is capable of carrying out mathematical and scientific calculations.

scientific notation A method of expressing large numbers so that there is no confusion about the number of digits, e.g. $2\,350\,000\,000$ is written as 2.35×10^9.

specific gravity The comparison of the weight of a liquid with an equal volume of distilled water.

sphygmomanometer A machine that is used to measure blood pressure.

spirometry The assessment of a patient's respiratory capacity.

standard administration set An intravenous fluid administration set that delivers 20 drops per millilitre of fluid.

standard form Expressing large numbers so that there is only one number in front of the decimal point, and the rest of the number is put in the form of a power of 10, e.g. $157\,000\,000$ can be written as 1.57×10^8.

statistics The information gained from collecting and analysing quantities of data.

statistical test A method for analysing and verifying the results of data collection.

subcutaneous Under the skin, such as in the administration of drugs that need to be absorbed slowly.

subtraction Minus or taking away one number from another, finding the difference between two numbers.

summary of product characteristics The information that is given by the manufacturer on the leaflets inserted into the packaging.

surface tension The effect of the attraction of molecules of a liquid to each other and to the sides of its container.

synthetic A substance made from artificial sources.

syringe driver A portable device used to deliver drugs via a small syringe.

syringe pump A device attached to a pole or rack used to deliver drugs using a large syringe.

Système International d'Unités' (SI units) An agreed standard for defining the measurement of physical properties such as mass, length and volume used in scientific practice.

systolic pressure The upper reading of blood pressure produced by the pressure of the blood on the arterial walls when the ventricles of the heart contract.

tachycardia A heart rate of over 100 beats per minute.

tidal volume The amount of air taken in and breathed out during each respiratory cycle.

total daily dose (TDD) The amount of drug calculated from a prescription that states the number of milligrams per kilogram per day.

TPR Temperature, Pulse and Respiration recordings are basic to any assessment of a patient.

tympanic membrane The correct name for the eardrum.

ulna The bone of the forearm that forms the elbow and is on the inside of the arm when the palm is facing upwards.

unfractionated Naturally sourced heparin from cows and pigs.

units A measurement of drug activity rather than drug weight or volume.

urinalysis The testing of urine to determine the presence of abnormalities.

variable In statistics this is the element of the research that can be changed or varies.

vial A container of powdered drug that has a synthetic rubber stopper.

vulgar fractions Common fractions where one number (numerator) is written over another (denominator), e.g. $\frac{7}{10}$.

Answer key

Chapter 1

WHAT DID YOU LEARN?
(a) 72 (b) 97 (c) 4504 (d) 15 (e) 1387 (f) 40 204 (g) 325 (h) 3891 (i) 64 (j) 10^9 (k) 19 (l) 27.

MORE 'TIME TO TRY' EXAMPLES

Number bonds 1–100, p. 7
(a) 30 (b) 75 (c) 53 (d) 12 (e) 87 (f) 49 (g) 81 (h) 38 (i) 54 (j) 67 (k) 27 (l) 43.

Addition, p. 8
(a) 169 (b) 798 (c) 398 (d) 379 (e) 599 (f) 995 (g) 888 (h) 998 (i) 296 (j) 696 (k) 894 (l) 799.

Addition – carrying over, p. 10
(a) 406 (b) 582 (c) 812 (d) 1181 (e) 560 (f) 741 (g) 1354 (h) 655 (i) 841 (j) 1287 (k) 542 (l) 1226.

Subtraction, p. 12
(a) 4 (b) 5 (c) 4 (d) 5 (e) 7 (f) 3 (g) 3 (h) 3 (i) 5 (j) 6 (k) 14 (l) 6.

Subtraction with borrowing, p. 14
(a) 24 (b) 39 (c) 16 (d) 36 (e) 59 (f) 56 (g) 87 (h) 38 (i) 193 (j) 557 (k) 280 (l) 340.

Multiplication, p. 18
(a) 70 (b) 0 (c) 351 (d) 308 (e) 388 (f) 2172 (g) 4656 (h) 1274 (i) 599 (j) 15 864 (k) 34 092 (l) 8715.

Multiplication, p. 20
(a) 33 524 (b) 46 624 (c) 56 236 (d) 11 808 (e) 15 778 (f) 19 505 (g) 7208 (h) 7144 (i) 21 682 (j) 29 326 (k) 19 995 (l) 21 423.

Division, p. 21–22
(a) 8 (b) 21 (c) 8 (d) 12 (e) 42 (f) 28 (g) 22 (h) 523 (i) 1935 (j) 357 (k) 354 (l) 185.

Chapter 2

WHAT DID YOU LEARN?
(a) (i) 2/3 (ii) 3/4 (iii) 3/8 (iv) 5/6 (v) 1/2 (vi) 1/3 (b) 3/4 (1 − 3/12) (c) 2/5 (d) 5 (find 1/4 and 1/3 of 12, then subtract the total from 12) (e) 37.6°C (39.1 − 1.5) (f) £61.31 (11.2 × 5.45).

MORE 'TIME TO TRY' EXAMPLES

Addition of fractions, p. 33
(a) 6/7 (b) 4/5 (c) 11/15 (d) 3/4 (e) 1 (f) 8/11.

Equivalent fractions, p. 35
1. (a) (the others = 1/7) 2. (a) (the others = 1/2) 3. (c) (the others = 2/3) 4. (b) (the others = 1/4).

Equivalent fractions, p. 37
(a) 1/3 (b) 4/21 (c) 7/32 (d) 12/13 (e) 1/9 (f) 1/3.

Equivalent fractions, p. 38
(a) 7/12 (b) 9/14 (c) 5/6 (d) 5/8 (e) 13/21 (f) 3/10.

Mixed numbers, p. 39
(a) $4\frac{3}{4}$ (b) $3\frac{7}{8}$ (c) $7\frac{2}{9}$ (d) $7\frac{1}{2}$ (e) $7\frac{3}{4}$ (f) $7\frac{4}{9}$.

Subtraction of fractions, p. 41
(a) 1/20 (b) 1/6 (c) 7/18 (d) 1/10 (e) 5/9 (f) 1/20.

Mixed numbers, p. 41
(a) $1\frac{1}{12}$ (b) 5/6 (c) $2\frac{13}{20}$ (d) $1\frac{4}{5}$ (e) 4/9 (f) $1\frac{1}{15}$.

Multiplication of fractions, p. 43
(a) 3/20 (b) 1/4 (c) 1/5 (d) $7\frac{1}{2}$ (e) $2\frac{6}{7}$ (f) 18/25.

Division of fractions, p. 44
(a) $3\frac{4}{7}$ (b) 1/2 (c) $5\frac{1}{2}$ (d) $2\frac{5}{8}$ (e) $2\frac{1}{25}$ (f) 9/14.

Addition and subtraction of decimal fractions, p. 47
(a) 3.86 (b) 11.01 (c) 25.422 (d) 1.13 (e) 2.88 (f) 3.89.

Multiplication of decimal fractions, p. 48
(a) 35 (b) 5700 (c) 314.2 (d) 14 900 (e) 34 500 000 (f) 175.3.

Multiplication of decimal fractions, p. 50
(a) 4.08 (b) 25.92 (c) 6.1755 (d) 17.752 (e) 15.1678 (f) 8.432.

Division of decimal fractions, p. 51
(a) 4.23 (b) 3.6761 (c) 0.0346 (d) 1.6522 (e) 4.302 225 (f) 20.08.

Division of decimal fractions, p. 53
(a) 2.00 (b) 2.03 (c) 25.60 (d) 12.60 (e) 0.50 (f) 27.56.

Chapter 3

WHAT DID YOU LEARN?

(a) cubic metre (b) litre (c) it is in working order, it is safe to use, it is accurate and you under-stand how it works (d) meniscus (e) 1.2 L (f) micro (g) kilogram (h) mass is constant, weight varies with the force of gravity (i) (i) 0.25 g (ii) 1700 mL (iii) 2000 mmol (iv) 1 330 000 micrograms (v) 4300 mg (vi) 0.25 m.

MORE 'TIME TO TRY' EXAMPLES

Page 70

(a) 2.754 kg (b) 1430 g or 1.43×10^3 g (c) 0.0035 kg or 3.5×10^{-3} kg (d) 1200 mL or 1.2×10^3 mL (e) 10 000 000 nanometres or 1.0×10^7 nanometres (f) 0.375 L or 3.75×10^{-1} L.

Chapter 4

WHAT DID YOU LEARN?

(a) 15 (b) 15.68 (c) the name given by the original manufacturer (d) the lower line of the meniscus should be held at eye level (e) pipette (f) body weight and body surface area (g) 186 mg (h) (i) 3 mL (ii) 3 tablets (iii) 2 tablets (iv) 2.5 mL (v) 4 tablets (vi) 5 mL.

MORE 'TIME TO TRY' EXAMPLES

Page 80
(a) 2 tablets (b) 2.5 mL (c) 2 tablets (d) 2 tablets (e) 15 mL (f) 3 tablets (g) 7.5 mL (h) 12 mL.

Page 82–3
1. (a) 320 mg (b) 315 mg (c) 14 mg (d) 770 mg. 2. (a) 462.5 mg (b) 82.5 mg (c) 350 mg (d) 285 mg.

Page 84
(a) 1.26 mg (b) 48 mg (c) 340 mg (d) 80 mg.

Page 88
(a) 0.25 mL (b) 1.5 mL (c) 1.5 mL (d) 0.25 mL (e) 1.8 mL (f) 4.6 mL (g) 0.8 mL (h) 3.5 mL. Did you notice the similarity of the two drugs that had to be reconstituted?

Chapter 5

WHAT DID YOU LEARN?

(a) 76 units (b) 30 units.   (d) 0.4 mL of 5000 units/mL (b) 1.8 mL of 5000 units/mL
(c) 0.6 mL of 5000 units/mL (d) 0.6 mL of 25 000 units/mL (e) 1.2 mL of 5000 units/mL
(f) 1 mL of 5000 units/mL.

MORE 'TIME TO TRY' EXAMPLES

Page 100
(a) 0.3 mL of 5000 units/mL (b) 0.3 mL of 10 000 units/mL (c) 0.7 mL of 5000 units/mL
(d) 0.8 mL of 10 000 units/mL (e) 0.48 mL of 25 000 units/mL (f) 0.8 mL of 5000 units/mL.

Page 104
(a) 74.5 (b) 100 (c) 74.5 g (d) 100 g.

Chapter 6

WHAT DID YOU LEARN?

(a) 20% (b) 4% (c) 0.43 (d) 0.05 (e) 54 (f) 52.5 pence (g) 1.74 L (1740 mL) (h) 25 (i) 4 L (j) 495 mL
(k) 1200 mL (1.2 L) (l) 1 mL (m) 2.5 mL (n) 100 g (o) 2.25 g.

MORE 'TIME TO TRY' EXAMPLES

Page 112
(a) 10% (b) 60% (c) 13.3% (d) 62.5% (e) 25% (f) 66.7% (g) 2% (h) 5% (i) 11/50 (j) 17/20 (k) 2/5
(l) 3/10 (m) 23/50 (n) 11/20 (o) 3/25 (p) 16/25.

Page 113–114
(a) 27.5 (b) 75 (c) 384.2 (d) 168.4 (e) 643.2 (f) 132 (g) £1.75 (h) £9.25 (i) £2.45 (j) £2.00
(k) £32.40 (l) £11.66.

Page 114
(a) 0.63 (b) 0.37 (c) 0.02 (d) 0.59 (e) 35% (f) 7% (g) 19% (h) 62%.

Page 118–119
(a) 50 g (b) 9 g (c) 0.5 g (d) 21 g (e) 2.5 mL (f) 30 mL (g) 5 mL (h) 3 mL (i) 3 g (j) 1 g (k) 20 mL
(l) 15 mL.

Page 123

(a) 50 mL (b) 100 mL (c) 0.25 mL (d) 0.05 mL (e) 9:18 (f) 4:14.

Chapter 7

WHAT DID YOU LEARN?

(a) A standard fluid administration set delivers 20 drops per mL. Rate 56 drops per minute.
(b) A blood administration set is needed because it has a filter chamber to remove particles from the blood; 28 drops per minute. (c) Check the prescription, the expiry date, for any damage to or condensation on the outer pack and that the fluid does not contain any crystals. (d) (i) 67 drops per minute (ii) 200 drops per minute (e) (i) 10 mg (ii) 12 hours (f) in millimetres

(g) $\dfrac{\text{length of fluid in mm}}{\text{infusion time in hours}} = \text{mm/h}$ (h) $\dfrac{\text{length of fluid in mm}}{\text{infusion time in 24 hours}} = \text{mm/24 h}$

MORE 'TIME TO TRY' EXAMPLES

Page 135

(a) 42 dpm (b) 67 dpm (c) 56 dpm (d) 125 dpm (e) 101 dpm (f) 33 dpm (g) 30 dpm (h) 48 dpm (i) 28 dpm.

Page 136

(a) 333 mL/hour (b) 167 mL/hour (c) 250 mL/hour.

Chapter 8

WHAT DID YOU LEARN?

(a) 60–80 beats per minute (b) 70 is the diastolic pressure (c) ventricular contraction (d) (i) three times a day (ii) once a day or daily (e) 750 mL (f) (i) 22 (ii) 1.9 m^2 (g) any two from fever, trauma, tissue repair, sepsis (h) (i) 8400 kJ (ii) 10 500 kJ

MORE 'TIME TO TRY' EXAMPLES

Page 162

Intake = 2500 mL IV + 230 mL orally = 2730 mL
Output = 1665 mL + 300 mL = 1965 mL
Balance = 2730 − 1965 mL = 765 mL positive balance
500 mL of 5% dextrose to be carried over.

Page 163

(a) 0.6 m^2 (b) 1.8 m^2 (c) 2.4 m^2 (d) 2.0 m^2.

Page 164

(a) 19, underweight (b) 34, obese (c) 33, obese (d) 27, overweight (e) 26, overweight

Chapter 9

WHAT DID YOU LEARN?

(a) The way in which the body's systems are in balance to maintain health (b) erythrocytes, white cells and platelets (c) 45% (d) fibrinogen, prothrombin (e) 20kJ (f) the test for nitrites will be positive (g) 21% (h) the sample should be taken from the *side* of the finger, *not* the tip.

Chapter 10

WHAT DID YOU LEARN?

(a) Measurements of frequency and demographic data (b) Methods section (c) Ethical permission from the appropriate body, patient consent (d) Bar chart (e) The region of a normal distribution curve where the convex curve changes to a concave curve (f) It divides the range into halves (g) 11, 17, 20, 29, 30, 36, 38, 43 (h) (i) $n = 8$ (ii) $\Sigma x = 224$ (iii) $\bar{x} = 28$.

Index

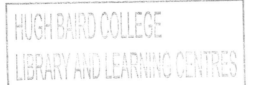